Brush—or Walk, Eat or Think—Your Headache Away!

Whatever you're doing for your headache, whether it's aspirin or the heavyweight prescription stuff, is probably doing you less good than you want—and doing nothing at all about *why* your head hurts.

Drawing on the latest research, Norman D. Ford shows you inexpensive, safe and effective ways to stop headaches, before or after they start.

Other Keats Titles of Related Interest

EIGHTEEN
NATURAL WAYS
TO BEAT
A HEADACHE

Norman D. Ford

Keats Publishing, Inc.   New Canaan, Connecticut

Eighteen Natural Ways to Beat a Headache is not intended as medical advice. Its intention is solely informational and educational. Please consult a medical or health professional should the need for one be indicated. The information in this book lends itself to self-help. For obvious reasons, the author and publisher cannot take the medical or legal responsibility of having the contents herein considered as a prescription for everyone. Either you, or the physician who examines and treats you, must take the responsibility for the uses made of this book.

Neither the author nor the publisher has authorized the use of their names, or the use of any of the material contained in this book, in connection with the sale, promotion or advertising of any product or apparatus. Any such use is strictly unauthorized and in violation of the rights of Norman D. Ford and Keats Publishing, Inc.

Library of Congress Cataloging-in-Publication Data

Ford, Norman D., 1921–
    Eighteen natural ways to beat a headache / Norman D. Ford.
      p.   cm.
    ISBN 0-87983-470-6
    1. Headache—Alternative treatment.   I. Title.   II. Title: 18
natural ways to beat a headache.
RB128.F568   1990
616.8'49106—dc20   90-4728
                                     CIP

Printed in the United States of America
KEATS PUBLISHING, INC.
27 Pine Street, New Canaan, Connecticut 06840

Contents

Acknowledgments

Most of the research behind this book was derived from some of America's most distinguished university medical centers and from such leading health advisory agencies as the National Institutes of Health, the American Heart Association, the National Academy of Sciences, and the Public Citizen Health Research Group. Virtually all of these studies support the validity and effectiveness of a multi-disciplinary approach to healing, and of the various alternative healing therapies described in this book.

So many sources were consulted in researching this book that it is impractical to acknowledge every one. However, I would like to acknowledge my debt to the research carried out by James Breneman M.D., Chairman, Allergy Committee, American Academy of Allergists; David E Bresler, Ph.D., director, Bresler Pain Center, Los Angeles; David R. Coddon, director, Headache Clinic, Mount Sinai Medical Center, New York; Seymour Diamond, M.D., director, Diamond Headache Clinic and National Migraine Foundation, Chicago; Arthur Elkind, M.D., director, Elkind Headache Clinic, Mount Vernon, New York; Arnold P. Friedman, M.D., founder, Montefiore Headache Unit, New York; Elmer E. Green, Ph.D., Menninger Foundation Biofeedback and Psycho-Physiology Center, Topeka, Kansas; Scott Haldeman, Ph.D., assistant clinical professor of neurology, University of California, Irvine; Robert S. Kunkel, M.D., director, Cleveland Clinic Headache Center; James Lance, M.D., University of New South Wales, Australia; Joan Millep, Ph.D., director, Atlanta Headache Clinic; Michael Moskowitz, M.D., Harvard University Medical School; Neil Raskin, M.D., professor of neurology, University of California, San Fran-

cisco; Joel R. Saper, M.D., director, Michigan Headache
and Neurological Institute; C. Norman Sheeley M.D., Pain
and Health Rehabilitation Center, La Crosse, Wisconsin;
Patricia Solbach, Ph.D., research psychologist, Menninger
Clinic, Topeka, Kansas; John E. Upledger, Ph.D., former
director, Unity Holistic Health Center, West Palm Beach,
Florida; American Association for the Study of Headache,
San Clemente, California; National Headache Foundation,
Chicago; National Migraine Foundation, Chicago; Califor-
nia Medical Clinic for Headache, Encino, California; Faulker
Headache Research Center, Boston; Houston Headache
Clinic, Houston; City of London Migraine Clinic, London,
England; UCLA Pain Management Center, Los Angeles.

Several short passages in Chapter 9 are quoted from the
author's companion book in this series, *Eighteen Natural
Ways to Beat the Common Cold*, Keats Publishing, Inc.,
1987.

1 The Drugless Way to Headache Relief

The snapping open of medicine cabinet doors as we reach inside for a pill to relieve a headache has become one of the most familiar sounds on the American scene.

Which is hardly surprising when you consider that TV ads bombard us with messages to reach for a pill for every ill. Altogether, we hand over more than two billion dollars annually for over the counter (OTC) and prescription drugs for headache relief.

Today, a huge multi-billion-dollar pharmaceutical and advertising industry has evolved, dedicated to conditioning us to believe that headaches can be cured only by a chemically active drug. For people who get only an occasional, simple tension headache, this is probably true. But what happens when two aspirin aren't enough?

All too many chronic headaches defy aspirin, and stronger painkillers are needed to dull the pain. Every drug is a two-edged sword; the pharmaceutical benefits are very often offset by adverse side effects. And the side effects of many headache drugs are so destructive that, at most headache clinics, the first step is to get new patients off all painkilling drugs, and then off any other non-essential medications, as swiftly as possible.

DRUGS MAY CAUSE MORE HEADACHES THAN THEY CURE

One reason is that so many chronic headache sufferers tend to take two or more medications on a daily basis. In 1984, at the New England Center for Headache in Greenwich, Connecticut (it has since moved to Stamford), a study was made on patients who took several different painkillers each day for their chronic headache pain. The drugs were gradually withdrawn altogether. After being drug-free for one month, 66 percent of the patients reported significantly fewer headaches and, after a second month, the number had grown to 81 percent.

At least half their headaches had been caused by the very drugs they were taking to try and relieve their headache pain.

Another reason why clinics immediately phase out painkilling drugs is that, even at recommended dosages, addiction to both OTC and prescription drugs can easily occur.

BREAKING THE BONDAGE OF DRUGS

According to a report in the National Headache Foundation's newsletter, fall, 1988, Arthur H. Elkind, M.D., director of the Elkind Headache Clinic in Mount Vernon, New York, stated at a national headache conference that many people with chronic headaches use excessive amounts of prescription and OTC medications for relief.

Drug dependency is common. Among medications that Dr. Elkind found most frequently abused were not only potent prescription drugs like ergotamine, barbiturates and

codeine, but OTC analgesics containing aspirin or acetaminophen, often in combination with caffeine.

We're not trying to exaggerate the risks of common
OTC headache medications. People generally know that
two aspirin will relieve most acute tension headaches within
half an hour without causing adverse side effects. Yet a
rule of thumb in most headache clinics is that if two
aspirin don't relieve a headache within thirty minutes,
taking more aspirin isn't likely to help.

A PILL FOR EVERY ILL

Most of us are so accustomed to assuming that a drug or
injection exists to provide instant relief for almost any kind
of pain, that we tend to see a drug solution for just about
every problem.

This has led most Americans to severely overestimate
the curative power of headache drugs. The cold facts are
that, for other than the occasional mild tension headache,
most anti-headache drugs are only 70 percent effective in
providing relief. And no really dependable drug exists for
treating cluster or menstrual migraine headaches.

Furthermore, studies have shown that approximately 33
percent of the benefits ascribed to headache medications
are due, not to any pharmaceutical action, but to the
placebo effect—to the patient's own belief in the drug's
ability to heal. When we subtract the healing power of the
placebo effect, it is only too apparent that drug therapy has
severe limitations of which most people are unaware.

A PHARMACOPOEIA OF HARSH AND
DANGEROUS DRUGS

Every drug, to some extent, is toxic to the human body,
so much so that doctors speak in terms of how well a
certain drug is tolerated. Even at recommended doses,

most drugs are mildly poisonous. For example, aspirin is so toxic that it can cause irritation or bleeding in the stomach and intestines, while continued use may erode the intestinal lining and form an ulcer. Common side effects of other headache drugs range from nausea to drowsiness, dizziness, confusion, bone loss, depression, vivid nightmares, insomnia, forgetfulness, breathing difficulties, rash and itching, hallucinations, blurred vision, dry mouth, kidney problems and even stroke.

However, virtually every headache specialist agrees that drugs may be essential for treating unusually stubborn cases of chronic headache. In severe cases of migraine and cluster headaches, a combination of drug and non-drug therapies may have to be used until the drugs can eventually be phased out.

But beyond these exceptions, the benefits of drug treatment often do *not* outweigh the risk of harm from adverse side effects. To some degree, most drugs are both carcinogenic and immunosuppressive, meaning that they may increase long-term risk of cancer and infections. Other headache drugs may increase risk of heart attack. It is widespread national concern about the disturbing side effects of these drugs that has renewed interest in non-drug ways to overcome headache.

All over America, the hazards and low efficacy of drug-focused headache treatment are promoting a renaissance for alternative health care therapies, a movement which is gaining increasing support from the health care professionals who staff the nation's headache and pain clinics.

HEADACHE CLINICS BEAT CHRONIC HEADACHES WITH DRUGLESS MEDICINE

Almost unknown to both doctors and the general public is the existance of some 25 medical clinics that specialize in headaches. In addition, several hundred medically operated pain clinics also treat headache pain. Many are associated with university medical centers and are manned by licensed health professionals from a variety of disciplines. These headache specialists have demonstrated a remarkable track record in achieving permanent relief from all types of headaches without drugs or other forms of mainstream medical treatment.

Although the clinics do employ drugs in extremely stubborn cases, the consensus of most headache specialists is that drugs are inappropriate for headache relief and that only natural, nonmedical therapies can permanently relieve most chronic headache pain.

Working with this philosophy, researchers at major headache clinics have made astonishing strides in developing natural, drugless therapies that relieve painful headaches, even when all other forms of treatment have failed. The anti-headache techniques used by these clinics employ do-it-yourself methods that almost anyone can use at home, usually without special know-how or equipment. The purpose of this book is to describe each of these anti-headache techniques so that you can begin to use them to treat your own headache pain.

STRESS IS THE UNDERLYING CAUSE OF MOST HEADACHES

Contributing to the success of most headache clinics is the growing recognition that stress is the underlying cause of the majority of headaches. This is hardly surprising since medical science now recognizes that virtually every disorder is stress-related, at least to some extent. Unresolved emotional stress is generally considered to be the underlying cause of at least 80 per cent of headaches, with the remainder being due to a variety of other forms of stress, ranging from the physical stress of noise or flickering lights, to the biological stress of low blood sugar.

Lack of funding, and difficulty in correlating stress to headaches in a laboratory setting, account for the paucity of documented evidence supporting the stress origin of headaches in medical journals. Compared to the $250 million awarded to research diabetes in 1989, the National Institute of Neurological Disorders and Stroke allotted a mere $1.4 million for headache research. Nonetheless, among headache specialists themselves, there is wide clinical acceptance of stress as the underlying cause of most headaches.

For example, *U.S. News* (July 31, 1989, page 4) begins its major coverage report on headaches by saying, "Stress has long been considered the principal cause of all headaches." And Arnold Fox, M.D. and Barry Fox, Ph.D., authors of *The Beverly Hills Diet*, recently advised in *Let's Live* Magazine (September 1989, page 59) that we should "start attacking the number one cause of headaches: stress."

Migraines are no exception. Discussing migraine trigger mechanisms, the Migraine Foundation of Toronto, Canada, states in its literature, "Migraine is triggered by precipitating or provoking factors—elements of stress, whether physical, emotional or situational that, given the predisposition, set off the actual headache process." The same literature notes that stress can consist of worry, anxiety, tension, emotional change, excitement, shock, repressed hostility, anger or depression, all arising from life situations.

Again, Dr. Seymour Diamond, director of the Diamond Headache Clinic and National Migraine Foundation, Chicago, stated recently that, "Our modern world is rampant with tension, frustration, anxiety, depression and repressed hostility, all of which can trigger headache pain. A multitude of chronic, recurring headaches are precipitated by stress."

And in his headache classic, *Headaches, The Drugless*

Way to Lasting Relief (Celestial Arts, 1987), Harry C. Ehrmantraut, Ph.D. states, "As a general rule, it is safe to say that a tension headache is precipitated by tension in the immediate life situation. This may arise from anger, aggravation, frustration, guilt or related emotional states."

Several authorities believe that marital stress is one of the most common causes of headaches. To confirm this, Rajan Roy, Ph.D., associate professor of social work and psychiatry at the University of Manitoba, studied 15 married couples. In each marriage, one partner suffered from recurrent tension or migraine headaches and all were experiencing marital stress. After a series of counseling sessions designed to reduce marital stress, 11 of the headache sufferers reported that their headaches were vastly improved.

Certainly, headaches can be provoked by drugs, illness, alcohol or other causes. But the prevailing opinion of most headache specialists is that the majority of headaches are provoked by negative emotions arising out of conflicts concerning job, money, marriage or similar life situations.

HEADACHES ARE A WHOLE PERSON DYSFUNCTION

Another reason that headache clinics have been eminently successful is that their treatment methods are based on the Whole Person or holistic approach. This is logical since almost all headaches begin with emotional stress that is translated into physiological mechanisms. Pain occurs as arteries in the head dilate. But the pain itself can only be experienced in the brain.

A headache is, therefore, a Whole Person phenomenon that involves the physical, mental, emotional, attitudinal, cognitive and even the nutritional and spiritual levels of the body-mind. Headache clinics respond to this Whole Person involvement by employing an array of alternative healing therapies which work on varying levels of body-mind function.

Doctors have attempted to duplicate the holistic approach by using a "background" drug as a daily prophylactic, and then using painkilling drugs whenever a headache occurs. As might be expected, this shotgun approach serves only to multiply side effects to the point where patients become increasingly depressed, helpless and dependent on drugs.

What most of us fail to recognize is that drugs often only duplicate tasks that the body-mind itself is entirely capable of doing in a normally healthy person.

In most cases, by using the natural therapies in this book, we may restore lost functions to the point where drugs are no longer needed. Our bodymind then becomes capable of taking over the job once more.

The Whole Person approach to healing is also known as holistic healing or holistic medicine. In medical science, its equivalent is behavioral medicine, a multi-disciplinary approach which employs multi-modal therapies. This means that behavioral medicine is administered by M.D.s. Although able to prescribe strong drugs should they be needed, behaviorial physicians prefer to minimize the use of pharmaceuticals, and most employ drugs only when absolutely essential. Much preferred are harmless, non-drug therapies such as acupuncture, acupressure, nutrition, massage exercise, heat and cold therapy, relaxation, biofeedback, creative imagery, stress management and cognitive positivism.

SELF-HELP FOR YOUR HEADACHE

Each of these natural therapies is widely used by headache and pain clinics and, of course, each is also freely available for anyone to use. By using a holistic approach, that is, using therapies that function on several different mindbody levels simultaneously, we can practice Behavioral Medicine on our own. By using several different natural therapies—for example, one physical, one nutritional and one cognitive—we can often intervene in our own headache with far greater success than by using drugs.

Natural therapies are classified as either active or passive. Active therapies are the core of behavioral medicine. By forcing us to take an active role in our own recovery, active therapies promote taking control of our lives and taking responsibility for our own wellness.

Among active therapies are attitudinal and cognitive therapies, exercise, relaxation, biofeedback, creative imagery, nutrition, heat and cold therapy, self-massage, acupressure, stretching and breathing techniques, identifying nutritional and environmental headache triggers, and do-it-yourself homeopathy and herbal medicine. Each encourages us to take action in response to our pain and stress and so to help ourselves.

This book can't exercise for you, relax for you, make images in your mind, or reprogram the beliefs that are causing your headaches. Behavioral medicine puts you in control and it's up to you to take an active role.

Among passive therapies are acupuncture, massage, homeopathy and herbal medicine prescribed by others as well as all drug medications. In each, something is *done to us* by a substance or by a person. While passive therapies can provide useful short-term relief, a holistic array of more active therapies is usually required to reverse the underlying cause of chronic headache pain.

HOLISTIC HEALING: THE NEW AGE MEDICINE

With all these options available, the drugless treatments you choose will be those that seem most appropriate for you and for your particular type of headache. Whichever you choose, we strongly recommend that you thoroughly read chapters 1, 2, and 3, which have to do with the attitudinal approach to anti-headache techniques.

For instance, the present chapter, Chapter 1, motivates you to minimize dependence on nonessential headache drugs. Chapter 2 urges you to obtain medical assurance that your headache is benign. And Chapter 3 describes how to gain power over your headache by becoming a medically informed layperson. Together, these chapters form the backbone of any Whole Person approach to permanent relief from chronic headache.

To play an active role in your own recovery from headaches—or any other dysfunction—you must know how to act and what to do. Thus the first step in practicing holistic healing is to acquire this know-how. By the time you have read and absorbed Chapters 1, 2, and 3, you will probably know more about headaches than your doctor does. Chapter by chapter, you should then read and absorb the remainder of this book. It is not a large book and a good reader can easily finish it in a single evening.

You will find that each chapter expands your knowledge of headaches and adds to the number of alternative therapies you can use.

We also very strongly urge that, as part of your holistic healing program, you include Anti-Headache Technique #17, **Liberate Yourself from Headaches With Cognitive Positivism.** For this is the *only* modality that can actually help rid us of the underlying cause of headaches.

Among other options, we recommend choosing one or more techniques from as many chapters as you can. Each chapter describes a group of therapies all of which function on a common approach. For instance, to relieve and banish chronic tension headache, you might choose these anti-headache techniques:

7-A, A Simple Stretching Technique.
12, Temperature Therapy for Speedy Relief.
14, Deep Relaxation With Muscle Tensing.
When these techniques, incorporating the physical and relaxation approaches, are coupled with Chapters 1, 2 and 3 and Technique #17, they offer a truly holistic approach.

To relieve and eventually banish chronic migraine, you might choose to employ these anti-headache techniques:

5, Headache Freedom Through Tryptophan Loading
6, Herbal Relief for Migraine Pain.
14 & 15, Deep Relaxation and Biofeedback.
These techniques use the nutritional, herbal and relaxation approaches. Together with Chapters 1, 2 and 3 and Technique #17, they also offer a truly holistic approach.

MINIMIZE DEPENDENCY ON NONESSENTIAL DRUGS

The focus of this chapter is on *minimizing dependency* on nonessential headache medications. It is not intended to dissuade you from taking drugs prescribed by your doctor, or drugs which may be essential to your health.

With this caveat in mind, the first step in freeing yourself from headaches is to take a cue from the headache clinics. Their prime concern is to get patients off painkillers as quickly as possible, and then off any other drugs.

If you are taking a prescription drug, or an OTC drug on your doctor's recommendation, or are under medical treatment for any reason at all, you must seek your doctor's approval and cooperation before reducing the dosage, and phasing out, any drug. Drugs prescribed for dysfunctions such as hypertension or heart disease may also precipitate chronic headaches. Your doctor may consider such drugs to be essential.

Even if your doctor does agree to phase out a drug, you

may have to do it under medical supervision because you may already be addicted to the drug.

GETTING FREE OF THE MEDICAL STRAITJACKET

If your physician is the type who overmedicalizes everything and attempts to solve all problems with drugs, you may want to seek a second medical opinion. Some physicians will prescribe a drug even when the problem is one for which drugs are not the best answer. When a side effect appears, they tend to view it as a brand new disease to be treated by prescribing yet another drug.

It would be wise to seek a second opinion about any decision to "manage" your headache with drugs on a long-term basis. This is especially important if you are taking a daily "background" drug and add a painkiller during attacks. It is all too possible that, far from being the best treatment for your condition, such drug management has been prescribed as the treatment least likely to provoke a litigation suit.

Side effects from "maintenance" drugs have turned many chronic headache sufferers into passive, helpless zombies. If you suspect you are being kept on a drug that you may not really need, you should seek a second medical opinion. Not all doctors are equally competent. Even within medicine, there is a choice of regimes for treating chronic headache. A second doctor may know of a less costly, less harmful, and more effective treatment of which your own doctor is unaware.

BACKLASH AGAINST PHARMACEUTICALS

One reason headache medications may fail to work is that the majority were originally developed for treating other diseases. While medical science has focused its efforts on finding a cure for killer diseases like cancer and heart disease, research into the causes and cure of headaches has been ignored. Primarily, this is because headaches are not usually life-threatening.

In 1987, the National Institutes of Health spent only $932,000 on headache research compared to over $500 million on heart disease. The result is that few drugs have been developed primarily for headache relief; and as far as curing chronic headaches goes, the other drugs don't appear to be getting the job done.

Headache drugs are classified as either abortive painkilling drugs or as prophylactic drugs.

Abortive Painkilling Drugs

Chief among these are the nonsteroidal anti-inflammatory drugs (NSAIDs) which inhibit synthesis of prostaglandins, hormone-like substances essential to the headache process. The principal NSAIDs include aspirin, acetaminophen and ibuprofen, all available OTC. These drugs work best on tension headaches.

Besides causing irritation or bleeding in stomach and intestines, continued use of aspirin may erode the intestinal lining and cause an ulcer. It can also impair blood coagulation, increase the tendency to bleed, lead to a higher risk of iron-deficiency anemia in younger women, and increase risk of a bleeding-type stroke. Nor are acetaminophen or ibuprofen panaceas. Each has a discouraging list of adverse side effects.

Once migraine begins, it can be stopped only by a powerful vasoconstrictor like ergotamine, a drug so fraught with side effects that it is prescribed only for severe migraine or cluster headache. Even then, it can be used only periodically. The steroid prednisone, occasionally prescribed to halt a cluster headache bout, has such a list of severe adverse side effects that it is used only when all else has failed.

Painkilling cocktails that often include codeine, tranquilizers or barbiturates are also commonly prescribed. All are addictive, and they are much overused. The analgesic lidocaine, another heart disease drug prescribed to relieve cluster headache, also carries a long list of adverse side effects.

Prophylactic Drugs

Prophylactic drugs are prescribed on a long-term basis to prevent headaches from occurring. Most carry risk of severe side effects and habitual dependency. Both beta blockers and calcium channel blockers are heart disease drugs, prescribed to reduce the severity and frequency of migraine and cluster headaches. Beta blockers work by blocking receptors in blood vessels to prevent constriction by norepinephrine. Calcium channel blockers achieve the same effect by blocking calcium uptake into muscles surrounding blood vessel walls. Both are addictive, may lead to constipation and drowsiness, and have a melancholy list of other adverse side effects.

Antidepressants are also prescribed when tension headaches seem due to depression or anxiety. They prevent uptake of serotonin into nerve cells, thus freeing existing serotonin to function as a neurotransmitter. Curiously, one of the many adverse side effects of these drugs is to heighten motivation for suicide, the very thing the drug is supposed to prevent. (Far superior results may be achieved through behavioral medicine by using a combination of **tryptophan loading** and **cognitive positivism**, techniques #5 and #17.

Yet another prophylactic drug prescribed for cluster headaches, lithium carbonate, poses a risk of kidney damage when employed for long-term use.

Among other drugs not to take for headaches are tranquilizers or muscle relaxants. Although they provide symptomatic relief of anxiety and tension, they intensify headache pain and often increase anxiety instead of relieving it.

Women may also want to avoid oral contraceptives. Roughly half of all women using the pill have complained of headaches after the first year. Powerful vasoconstrictors, oral contraceptives have been known to cause migraine accompanied by symptoms so severe that medical attention has been necessary. Headaches are also a common side effect of nitroglycerine and many other drugs.

This book will bring readers to the following conclusions:

1. Most drugs merely mask symptoms. Not a single drug can remove the underlying cause of most headaches, which is unresolved emotional stress.

2. Any therapy that does not use drugs offers enormous advantages over therapies that involve drug use.

ESCAPING THE DRUG TRAP

Assuming you are taking one or more OTC medications, which were not prescribed by a physician, the choice to stop using them is entirely up to you.

Before continuing to take any type of drug, you may want to ask yourself these questions:

Why am I taking this medication?

Is it really necessary and do I really need it?

What would happen if I did not take it?

What alternative therapies might be more effective, less costly, and free of destructive side effects? For example, before continuing to take a tranquilizer, have you considered such alternatives as exercise, deep breathing or deep relaxation—all much more effective, safer and cheaper than any drug?

These questions are not intended to discourage you from seeing a doctor, or from taking any drug that is really necessary. Obviously, some people are entirely unsuited to any form of therapy but drugs.

The idea is to get you thinking about stopping any drug that is not really needed. It is essential to try to minimize intake of every type of drug, because drugs may inhibit the effectiveness of natural therapies. Again, if you are taking a drug, it is difficult to assess the effects of behavioral medicine.

Meanwhile, if you must take drugs:

• Always take as few as possible.

• Ask for the minimum effective dosage for the shortest period of time.

BEAT HEADACHE MISERY WITHOUT USING DRUGS

Doctors are under tremendous pressure by drug manufacturers to place as many people as possible on lifelong maintenance drugs. All too often, both doctors and patients fail to realize that long-term use of headache drugs can lead to helplessness, hopelessness, depression and anxiety. In turn, these negative emotions merely exacerbate headache pain.

In reality, virtually all the functions achieved by drugs can also be achieved by using natural, drugless therapies instead. For example, drugs attempt to stop headache pain by intervening in bodily processes that are normally controlled by the involuntary nervous system. Most doctors consider that anything controlled by the involuntary nervous system is beyond our personal control. But behavioral medicine has effectively smashed this cherished belief by demonstrating that we can gain indirect control of several of the most important body functions involved in the headache process. In some cases, the techniques in this book may seem so indirect that it is like putting on a wool hat to warm the feet (actually one of the most effective ways to keep the feet warm). In headache therapy, by warming the hands and feet, we can draw blood away from the head and forestall a migraine attack.

CONTROL YOUR HEADACHE WITH NATURAL THERAPIES

It may be difficult at first to see that by creating an upbeat attitude, Chapters 2 and 3 actually put you in direct control of your headache. As you are transformed from a passive headache victim to a confident, medically-informed layperson, any tendencies toward helplessness, hopelessness, depression or anxiety should swiftly fade away. You learn that drugs are not the only way to overcome headaches and you become motivated to take an active role in your own recovery.

In Chapter 5, you learn to control foods that may be triggering your headache. You learn how to control low blood sugar. You learn how to control the migraine process with vitamins and minerals. And you learn how to control an important painkilling neurotransmitter in the brain by manipulating certain foods.

Chapter 6 reveals how to control headaches with a painkilling herb available in most health food stores, and how to control your headache through homeopathy.

Chapter 7 is filled with natural therapies that give you control over the diameter of your arteries and over defusing stress, anxiety and depression. You also learn how to control release of the brain's natural morphine-containing opiates that block headache pain from being experienced.

There are breathing techniques that can stop a migraine or cluster headache within minutes. And easy stretching techniques put you in control of chronic tension headaches.

In Chapter 8 you learn to use relaxation and biofeedback to gain control of your own involuntary nervous system. Through creative imagery you also learn how to mobilize your own body's placebo effect. Research has shown that, through the placebo effect, people with a strongly positive attitude recover 25–33 percent faster from *any* kind of ailment, disease or dysfunction from a minor headache to major surgery.

Again, through positivism, Chapter 9 helps you to gain direct control over your negative beliefs, thoughts and emotions—the underlying causes of almost all headaches. By controlling your thoughts, you can control your feelings—and can work toward feeling terrific all of the time.

Finally, Chapter 10 shows you how to take direct control of your life by helping you build a headache-free lifestyle.

FINDING YOUR WAY OUT OF THE DRUG JUNGLE

The trouble with relying on drugs to relieve headache pain is that their painkilling effect steadily loses power, forcing the sufferer to take ever-stronger painkillers with increasingly potent side effects. As these new, stronger drugs also continue to lose effectiveness, chronic headache victims are typically shuttled from one specialist to another, none of whom can find anything wrong. All too often, they are finally told by their own doctor, "There is nothing more that modern medicine can do. You'll just have to learn to live with your headache."

By showing that there are, indeed, many things that can be done to relieve headache pain, behavioral medicine offers new hope and optimism to all who are trying to find their way out of the drug jungle.

A cautionary note: While these natural therapies have been used with considerable success by a number of headache and pain clinics, there is, of course, no guarantee that any one therapy is going to work for everyone, or in every case every time. All we can say is that these methods have been reported to be successful at least 50 percent of the time. Naturally, if a therapy does not appear to work for you, you should switch to another alternative healing modality.

2 When to Seek Medical Help For Your Headache

Every year, tens of thousands of Americans mistakenly believe that their headache is due to a brain tumor or other serious disease. Records show that when this possibility is ruled out, almost every patient shows a significant and immediate improvement.

Anxiety worsens all headaches. By obtaining medical assurance that your headache is benign, you can work wonders in lessening anxiety. The relief that this news brings is often the biggest single step toward headache recovery. Furthermore, those who visit a headache or pain clinic are often delighted to learn that they can improve their condition while, at the same time, being weaned from drugs.

OBTAINING MEDICAL ASSURANCE THAT YOUR HEADACHE IS BENIGN

The remainder of this chapter covers how to go about seeking medical evaluation and the best ways to obtain it.

All headaches fall into one of two classes: disease-related or benign. The natural drugless therapies in this book are for use exclusively with benign headaches. So before reading on, it's important to make absolutely *certain* that your headaches really are benign. If your headaches are disease-related, you must seek medical advice and you should refrain from using any of the techniques in this book unless you have your physician's specific approval.

If you have been experiencing tension or migraine headaches for years, and the symptoms are not worsening, there probably isn't any urgent need for a medical checkup. A thorough evaluation by a headache clinic may cost $250–$500, and may be unnecessary for most people who suffer from a well-established pattern of chronic headaches. Only if symptoms are worsening, or if the pain is becoming unbearable and interfering with your work or family or social life, would you normally need to think about consulting a headache clinic.

Most of the therapies described in this book are similar or identical to those used by the majority of headache clinics. However, if you have any reason to think that you may require medical treatment, you should see your doctor or arrange to visit a headache clinic without delay.

Likewise, if you have any anxiety about your health and your headaches, you should arrange for a medical examination. Preferably this should be at a headache clinic. Or failing that, at a pain clinic or by a doctor who is experienced in headaches.

CHOOSING A HEADACHE OR PAIN CLINIC

Approximately 25 headache clinics exist in the U.S. The best are usually branches of major medical centers or universities, offer a multi-disciplinary (Whole Person) approach, and are staffed by specialists representing an array of disciplines, such as internists, neurologists, psychiatrists, physical therapists, and counselors. Other clinics may be operated by individual doctors with varying capabilities. It's best to seek a certified facility.

While most can be depended on for an expert diagnosis, smaller clinics may not offer the same wide option of alternative therapies as large, multi-disciplinary clinics. To help evaluate a clinic, check on the credentials of the staff and ask to see if they are board-certified in their field.

Most of America's several hundred pain clinics are also capable of diagnosing headaches, but not all specialize in headache treatment. Although the clinic itself may offer a multidisciplinary approach to pain relief, the headache department may offer only a single discipline. By comparison, virtually all bona fide headache clinics prefer a nondrug approach with emphasis on relaxation and biofeedback training, nutrition, massage, counseling and stress management. While some clinics accept patients without referral, others may require that you be referred by your doctor.

The average physician is probably quite capable of determining whether your headaches are disease-related or benign, but may not be as adept at diagnosing your headache *type*, and so may prescribe an inappropriate medication. The average doctor is also often unaware of the alternative, nondrug therapies used by most headache clinics, and will tend to rely upon drugs.

It is fairly common, in fact, for headache clinics to discover a misdiagnosis by a family doctor, who has also prescribed the wrong medication. When the medication is corrected and the patient introduced to other therapies, some patients are able to end their headaches in a short time.

How long does it normally take for a headache clinic to end chronic headaches permanently? That depends. In very stubborn cases, clinics may only be able to reduce the pain to manageable levels.

By contrast, benign chronic headaches can occasionally be permanently ended by a single therapy. But it's safest not to expect a magic bullet. Most clinics employ a holistic array of therapies that work on body, mind and belief system simultaneously. By working together synergistically, each reinforcing the other, a selection of these therapies can typically be expected to eliminate chronic migraine headaches in from 5 to 12 weeks.

WHEN SHOULD YOU SEEK MEDICAL HELP FOR YOUR HEADACHE?

If you have any of the following symptoms, seek medical care *immediately*. If circumstances warrant, call an ambulance or have someone take you to the nearest hospital emergency room.

A headache associated with loss of movement on one side of the body.

A new, sharp, sudden, severe or stabbing headache that causes you to stop whatever you're doing.

A headache in which it is painful to bend the head forward and which may also be accompanied by fever, drowsiness, altered moods, nausea or light hurting the eyes.

A very severe headache that is new or unusual.

Any headache that occurs after a recent head or neck injury.

Any headache accompanied by dizziness, double vision or loss of memory.

Any headache that makes you feel ill, especially if you have difficulty finding the right words or in calculating.

You're over 50 and have a headache associated with

fever, eyesight problems, weight loss and a pain on one side of the jaw while chewing.

You have a sudden, explosive, thunderclap-type headache for the first time, especially if it is the worst headache of your life.

Your headache is associated with fever, convulsions or loss of consciousness.

Symptoms such as these could indicate such serious disorders as a ruptured aneurysm or a blood clot in a carotid or inter-cranial artery, a stroke, meningitis, a brain tumor, an epileptic seizure or temporal arteritis.

Brain tumors are actually quite rare and you are very unlikely to have one. A brain tumor headache becomes progressively worse, and is accompanied by vomiting and severe disturbances of vision, speech or personality. Even then, many cases can be treated by surgery or radiation.

While the following headache symptoms don't require *immediate* attention, you should see a doctor as soon as possible.

You're over 50 and have a headache for the first time.

A young child has a persistently recurring headache.

Your headache symptoms differ from preceding patterns, especially if associated with pain in an eye or ear.

A headache is frequent, severe and sudden.

A headache occurs almost daily.

A headache occurs during or immediately after exercise, lovemaking or a bowel movement; or when coughing, bending, straining or sneezing.

A headache begins when you wake up from a sound sleep.

A headache is so severe that you must take pain relievers daily or almost daily.

You experience any sudden deteriorating change in headache pattern.

You have a headache that grows progressively severe as time goes on and is always in the same location.

A headache lasts 12 hours or more without dissipating.

A headache is accompanied by numbness in an arm or leg.

You have always experienced migraine pain on one side of the head and now it shifts to the other side.

For the first time you have a headache accompanied by visual disturbances, or weakness of one side of a body area, or dizziness or speech disorders.

A headache recurs in a similar pattern day after day, under the same circumstances, at the same time, in the same location, and for the same duration.

A headache is new and persistent when previously you had no headaches.

A headache is persistent and incapacitating.

A headache cannot be numbed by the strongest over-the-counter medications.

While such symptoms could be less urgent indicators of the same disorders described earlier, they could also be due to infections such as the Epstein-Barr virus. Requiring less urgent medical treatment are headaches due to a sinus infection, eyestrain, a deviated septum or hypertension.

ALMOST ALL HEADACHES ARE BENIGN

The message of this chapter is that if you have symptoms of any disease-related headache, you should consult a physician or headache clinic. Only after you have been assured that your headache is benign should you practice any of the therapies in this book. And for that also, you are advised to consult a doctor first.

The symptoms for disease-related headaches described in this chapter apply to fewer than two percent of all headaches. Which means that more than 98 percent of all headaches are benign. Although painful and, at times, even debilitating, a benign headache is not due to any underlying disease or disorder. Nor will it directly pose a threat to your health.

These caveats dispensed with, the remainder of this book is about benign headaches, and how you can help prevent and overcome these disorders without resorting to either OTC or prescription drugs.

3 Understanding Headache Dynamics Is the Key to Relief

The more you learn about the basics of headache mechanisms, the less reason you have to fear headaches. A sound knowledge of the headache process can give you a powerful feeling of being in control of not only your headache but of your health and life as well.

No longer do you need to feel a victim of random attacks . . . or totally dependent on drugs.

GAINING POWER OVER YOUR HEADACHE BY BECOMING MEDICALLY INFORMED

Choosing to learn more about the headache process is the first step in using behavioral medicine, the medical extension of holistic healing. By simply understanding how your body-mind produces a headache, you will find yourself transformed from a passive, helpless headache victim into a confident, medically informed layperson ready to take an active role in overcoming your chronic headache.

Before you can intervene successfully in your headache, you must know which type of headache you have. Basically, there are two types, disease-related headaches and benign recurrent headaches.

Disease-related headaches were discussed in Chapter 2. If you have not already done so, you should read Chapter 2 now. Disease-related headaches may require immediate medical attention. The natural therapies in this book are *not* intended for people with disease-related headaches.

All other headaches are classified as benign.

Benign Recurrent Headaches

Two types of benign headaches exist: Muscle Contraction Headaches and Vascular Headaches.

Muscle Contraction or Tension Headaches account for the vast majority of headaches. Almost invariably they are caused by unresolved emotional stress which is translated through the fight-or-flight response into abnormal contraction of the shoulder, neck and scalp muscles. There are two classes of tension headaches.

Acute tension headaches are isolated headaches generally caused by stress. They can normally be relieved by OTC drugs or by natural therapies and medical help is seldom required.

Chronic tension headaches persist day after day without relief. Many chronic tension headaches are linked to anxiety and depression and can continue without letup for years. Drugs serve only to temporarily relieve symptoms. The only treatment that really works is **Cognitive Positivism** (Technique #17).

Some variants of tension headaches are combination tension-vascular headaches, including exertion headaches, and those associated with temporomandibular joint syndrome, or TMJ. These are discussed after the next section, on vascular headaches.

Vascular Headaches. Usually caused by unresolved emotional stress, which triggers the fight-or-flight response, these headaches are set in motion by a complex series of biochemical reactions that cause changes in blood vessels and in blood flow in the head.

Whether or not the fight-or-flight response sets off a muscle contraction headache, or a vascular headache, or no headache at all, appears to depend on an individual's personal neurological chemistry. Headache specialists prefer to say that one person may have a biochemical predisposition to tension headaches, for example, while another may have a predisposition to migraine headaches. In either case, the headache mechanism is set in motion when the fight-or-flight response is invoked.

The most common vascular headache is migraine, which has several variants: some exertion headaches; hangover; caffeine withdrawal; ice cream; hunger; and menstrual headaches. Cluster headaches are another type of vascular headache.

Migraine Headaches. There are two distinct types of migraine headaches.

Classic Migraine Headache in which the headache is preceded by a spectacular "aura," consisting of visual disturbances and distortions of senses and perceptions. Usually, these symptoms last from 10–30 minutes, sometimes up to one hour, before they fade away and the headache begins.

Only 20 percent of migraines are classic; the remainder are common migraines.

Common Migraine Headache in which the prodromal (aura) sensations are so diffuse that they often amount to no more than a vague feeling of fogginess and irritability. As these uncertain symptoms disappear, the severe throbbing pain of migraine begins.

Cluster Headaches. The other type of vascular headache is the dreaded cluster. Two different types of clusters have been identified.

- Episodic or Cyclic Cluster Headache recurs in a pattern. Four of every five cluster headaches are episodic. They usually occur in bouts (hence the name cluster), after which they disappear for a year or more before returning in another bout. Breathing pure oxygen can shorten 70 percent of cluster headaches 70 percent of the time. But it is inconvenient to carry an oxygen bottle around.
- Chronic Cluster Headaches are acute attacks that recur regularly without remission for a period of one year or more. They are difficult to prevent pharmaceutically and, though they can be treated with analgesics, the attack is often over before the painkiller has begun to work.

COMBINATION AND VARIANT HEADACHES

Approximately ten percent of people with chronic tension headaches experience an occasional migraine headache superimposed on the tension headache. At this time, their headache worsens and they feel the throbbing pain of a vascular headache in addition to the steady, dull ache of the tension headache.

This is believed to be due to a vascular component in

some tension headaches. Most combination headaches are free of aura displays but the symptoms of common migraine are superimposed on those of the tension headache. Such headaches are best treated as migraines until the migraine ends, at which time therapy should be resumed for the tension headache.

Sexual Headaches. Another combination variant is the Benign Sexual Headache. The headache appears in two ways: either as a steady ache starting a few minutes before orgasm; or as a pulsating headache that suddenly begins at or near climax. Either type of headache may persist for several hours.

Headache specialists have suggested that sexual headaches are due to a combination of muscle contraction and blood vessel dilation set off by a sudden increase in blood pressure resulting from the excitement and exertion. These headaches usually appear in middle-aged men who are overweight, sedentary and mildly hypertensive. After several months, they often disappear. Though physically harmless, a benign sexual headache can have a traumatic effect on a person's love life.

Since a sexual headache could be confused with a stroke, you should consult a physician to confirm that the headache is actually benign. Your doctor may suggest a combination of exercise coupled with gradual weight loss to effectively lower blood pressure and overcome the headache.

TMJ Headaches. A fairly common variant of tension headache is due to the TMJ or Temporomandibular Joint Syndrome. People with deep anxiety often grind their teeth while asleep. This creates a painful spasm in face, neck and jaw muscles, particularly in the temporomandibular joint at the hinge of the jaw. Nerves refer the pain up to the forehead where it manifests as a headache in the temples and behind or below the eyes. A sign that a headache may be due to the TMJ syndrome is tenseness in the jaw on awakening and a feeling that the teeth have been tightly clenched.

The TMJ syndrome can often be relieved through relaxation or biofeedback training (Chapter 8). Otherwise, one should consult a dentist, preferably a member of the American Association of Oral and Maxillofacial Surgeons. Dentists are generally more aware of the TMJ process than doctors, and most are equipped to solve the problem.

They do so by making a light acrylic splint to be worn between the teeth while asleep. By making the teeth mesh correctly, the splint relaxes the jaw muscles so that they remain unstressed throughout the night. This usually stops the headaches.

Menstrual Migraines. In diagnosing a benign headache, it is helpful to know that both tension and migraine headaches are twice as common in women as men. By comparison, 19 of every 20 cluster headache sufferers are male.

Seventy percent of migraine sufferers are women in their childbearing years. In 60 percent of women migraineurs, the attacks occur during the week preceding, or during, menstruation. Other women experience migraine at the midpoint of the menstrual cycle, during ovulation. Migraines related to the menstrual cycle are often called menstrual migraines.

Menstrual migraines usually end by the third month of pregnancy, and the arrival of menopause liberates most women from further migraines. These clues indicate that migraine is related to hormone instability. And, indeed, taking estrogen or birth control pills *can* increase the frequency and intensity of migraine in women.

Most headache specialists believe that migraines are due to an inherited biochemical or hormonal imbalance. As a result, migraines tend to run in families. Thus children may experience migraines at a quite early age. Symptoms are similar to those in adults. Any child with migraine

should be checked by a pediatrician to rule out the possibility of a disease-related headache.

Efforts to define a migraine personality have been un-
successful, but many migraineurs seem to have low blood
pressure, flexible arteries, cold hands, low blood sugar and
unusually sensitive nerves. Women may experience menstrual irregularities. Classic migraineurs tend to be perfec-
tionists, compulsively tidy and well-groomed, and may
speak in hurried phrases. Many high achievers have been
migraine sufferers.

Our personal observations indicate that the majority of
people who suffer chronic headaches, both tension and
migraine, are unable to handle stress in a relaxed way.
Perhaps this is one reason why headaches are more common in younger than in older people. Headaches are most
prevalent in women aged 20 to 30 and in men aged 30 to
40.

UNLOCKING THE SECRETS OF HEADACHE PATHOLOGY

Until recently, it was thought that headaches were caused
by muscle contraction or by changes in blood vessels.
Now we know that these phenomena are merely part of a
deeper and more complex biochemical and neurological
process. There is also a growing recognition that the underlying cause of nearly all benign headaches is unresolved
emotional stress.

We have now learned that most headaches develop in
four separate stages, and that each stage has its specific
treatment requirements, whether by drugs or by behavioral
medicine. Drugs or natural therapies that work in Stage 2,
for example, are often not effective in Stages 3 or 4; and
only nondrug therapies are effective in Stage 1.

By learning about these stages, you can easily recognize

the stage which your headache has reached. You can then choose the most appropriate anti-headache technique for that stage.

STAGE 1

Stage 1 is common to all three types of headaches: tension, migraine and cluster headaches.

New information emerging from the research frontiers of medical science is revealing that the underlying cause of most chronic, recurrent headaches is chronic, recurrent stress. As previously explained in Chapter 1, at least 80 percent of all headaches are believed to be set off by unresolved emotional stress.

Our lives today are filled with potentially stressful events capable of triggering a painful headache. Conflicts concerning job, family, money and relationships; noise and constantly ringing telephones; traffic jams and waiting in line, long tiring drives on the freeway . . . the modern world is filled with potentially headache-provoking situations.

However, stress is caused by the way we react to a situation, not by the situation itself. Most migraine sufferers characteristically overreact to events they perceive as immediately threatening or disturbing, while most tension headache sufferers tend to be anxious and worried about upcoming events.

We can understand how headaches begin when we realize that every feeling (emotion) is preceded by a thought. Whenever we think a positive thought, we experience a positive emotion such as love, joy, hope, compassion, contentment or gratitude. Whenever we think a negative thought, we swiftly experience a negative emotion such as fear, anger, hostility, resentment, guilt, frustration, envy or anxiety.

Positive thoughts arise from positive beliefs held in our

belief system while most negative thoughts arise because we continue to hold outdated conditioned beliefs that we acquired in the past and that are no longer valid or appropriate.

The human mind has been aptly described as a biological computer. Information about the world around us is fed into the brain's interpretive center, where it is matched with data held in our belief system. After perceiving the input data through a filter of our beliefs, our interpretive center responds by placing a thought in our mind.

For example, if we have just learned that a friend has been given a promotion that we expected to get, this information is matched in our belief system with associations from the past. Depending on the beliefs in our data banks, our mind could choose a positive, loving thought that makes us feel glad for our friend's success. Or it could choose the negative thought that considering all the hard work we'd put in over the years without recognition, *we* should have been chosen for the promotion instead.

If a positive thought arose, it would immediately provoke a positive feeling. And a negative thought would provoke a negative feeling. We experience our feelings in the limbic area of the brain that surrounds the hypothalamus and pituitary glands. These glands scan every feeling we experience.

The Healing Power of Positive Beliefs

Positive emotions are recognized as friendly, which is a signal for the glands to turn on the body's relaxation response. This is a calm, relaxed state of serenity and peace. The parasympathetic branch of the autonomic nervous system takes over and maintains routine metabolism. Muscular tension melts away and negative thoughts and feelings disappear. The heart rate drops, blood pressure falls, respiration slows, oxygen consumption is reduced and immunocompetence soars.

As we enter the relaxed alpha state, brainwave frequency drops to 8 to 13 cycles per second. We feel comfortable and relaxed and we experience a delightful state of ease and wellness in which headaches are rarely experienced.

By contrast, the hypothalamus and pituitary glands recognize all negative emotions as threatening or unfriendly. Whenever confronted with a negative feeling, even a mildly negative feeling like boredom or uncertainty, these twin glands turn on all or part of the body's fight-or-flight response.

Negative Beliefs as a Cause of Headache

Fight-or-flight is a hair-trigger response that evolved in primitive times to prepare the body to meet imminent physical danger. The sympathetic nervous system, the emergency branch of the autonomous nervous system, takes over and all systems are Go. The adrenal glands squirt hormones into the blood stream to speed up body functions. Nerve fibers signal the smooth muscles to constrict every artery and arteriole. Blood pressure shoots up, and blood is shunted from the digestive system to the brain and muscles. Glycogen (sugar) is released from the liver, filling our muscles with energy and tensing them for action. Meanwhile, the clotting ability of blood platelets increases in preparation for a possible wound.

The problem is that this response, a legacy from pre-caveman days, can be turned on by any kind of feeling that the hypothalamus and pituitary glands interpret as negative. All too many people have such inappropriate belief systems that a letter from the IRS can trigger the same emergency state that their ancestors would have experienced on being confronted by a saber-toothed tiger.

If we act out the fight-or-flight response by either fighting or fleeing (or by jogging, bicycling, briskly walking or doing pushups), we release the pent-up muscular tension and the other stress mechanisms swiftly fade away. But if, as is so often true in modern society, physical action is impossible, we remain tensed-up and uncomfortable and we live through the day in a state of distress.

Trying to repress a negative emotion, which means concealing or burying or denying our discomfort, only intensifies our stress. Many people live in a continuously low-level emergency state with all their stress mechanisms constantly simmering. It is these stress mechanisms—the release of adrenal hormones, tensing of muscles, and heightened clotting ability of the platelets—that set off the remaining stages in the headache process.

Psychological Origin of Physical Disorders

In Stage 1, our negative thoughts are translated into physiological states that can produce an ulcer, a heart attack, a stroke, an infection, cancer or a headache. In fact, medical science now recognizes that virtually every disease or dysfunction has a stress component. Which disorder we actually get depends on our genetic makeup. If our coronary arteries are prone to spasm, a stress mechanism can set off unstable angina and a heart attack. If we are prone to headaches, we may get a tension, a migraine, or a cluster headache. The type we get will be the one to which our body chemistry makes us most prone.

Although Stage 1 is the cause of most headaches, drugs or medical treatment can be of little help at this level. This emphasizes once again that most drugs merely serve to palliate symptoms while the root cause of disease may be eliminated by drugless behavioral medicine.

The most effective single step that most chronic headache sufferers can take is to let go of all beliefs that cause or intensify headaches and to replace them with new beliefs that minimize headaches and that engender high-level wellness.

One can only guess at how many millions of migraine headaches are suffered annually by people who continue to believe ''I will never forgive so-and-so because of what he or she did to me.'' Such a destructive belief is a ''hair trigger'' which can set off a headache on the slightest provocation.

Meanwhile, we estimate, every year at least several thousand migraineurs achieve immediate and permanent liberation from their headaches when they learn to forgive everyone whom they believe may have harmed them.

Through behavioral medicine, we can eliminate most stress, and thereby end most headaches, by changing the way we perceive events, so that instead of seeing them as threatening, we see them as neutral or friendly. Chapter 9 describes how to absorb into your belief system all new beliefs that lessen headache pain, and to drop all those that intensify headache pain.

STAGE 2

In this intermediate stage, stress mechanisms cause changes to blood vessels and to blood flow in the head. In Stage 2, each headache type follows a separate path.

Tension Headaches

As energy pours into muscles throughout the body, tensing them for emergency action, the shoulders, neck, scalp and facial muscles also contract. The trapezius muscle, which connects the shoulder, neck and collarbone, may contract into a knot.

In the neck area, muscles, nerves and arteries are all closely packed. Prolonged tension in the muscles of shoulders and neck excites neural pathways that refer pain impulses up to the sweatband area for a second phase of muscular contraction.

These nerve impulses control the synthesis of prostaglandin, a hormonelike substance released by the immune system in response to stress. Prostaglandin immediately induces contraction in the smooth muscles of blood vessels in the headband area, as well as making nerve endings in these blood vessels exquisitely sensitive to pain.

Prostaglandin synthesis is an essential step in muscle contraction headaches. To a lesser extent it also occurs in the vascular headache process. When this step is blocked by intervention, tension headache pain cannot be perceived.

Nowhere is constriction more evident than in the occipital artery, which supplies a network of arterioles that radiate out behind the ears and into the headband area of the scalp. In a desperate attempt to bring in more blood and oxygen, these blood vessels burst into a vigorous dilation.

The overall effect is to dilate blood vessels in a wide band around the head that includes the temples, forehead and hatband area.

All is now ready for the headache to begin in Stage 3.

Classic Migraine

Roughly one-fifth of all migraine headaches are the classic type, meaning that they are preceded by a series of prodromal sensations, commonly known as an *aura*. Appearing before the eyes as a dazzling display of star bursts, zigzag lines and patches of blackness, these visual disturbances are dreaded by most migraine sufferers. After 10 to 30 minutes, the aura activity ends and the migraine pain hits.

Besides visual disturbances, aura symptoms may include numbness in an arm or leg; a slurring of words or similar speech impediment; acute sensitivity to glaring, flashing or flickering light; bizarre changes in smell, taste, or touch; cold hands; weakness or numbness in one side of the body; tingling in legs, arms, hands or face; nasal congestion; watery eyes and difficulty in focusing eyes; distorted perception; and restlessness or confusion.

Some migraine sufferers worry that prodromal visual disturbances may be due to a detached retina. Very rarely is this so. Moreover, some people experience aura symptoms without ever experiencing any migraine pain. This is known as a migraine equivalent. Here again, the symptoms are often confused with those of a transient ischemic attack which may herald a stroke. However, a true migraine equivalent is not associated with a stroke.

Aura symptoms are purely neurological in origin and are set off by a "nerve storm" that slowly moves across the brain from front to back. This phenomenon, discovered in the 1980s by Jes Oleson and Martin Lauritzen, two University of Copenhagen researchers, explains the aura effect in terms of a partial shut-down of cerebral blood circulation.

As the aura commences, the Danish researchers discovered, there is a 25 percent drop in blood flow at the back of the brain. In a wavelike motion, this depression moves from the back of the brain to the front. As it moves, it activates the visual cortex and sets off neurological mechanisms that produce the aura effect in front of the eyes.

Although the wave motion is neurological and emanates from the central nervous system, the reduced blood flow is actually created by the opening of blood vessels called shunts. These carotid shunts bypass incoming blood from the carotid arteries and carry it directly back into the veins.

Normally, blood from the carotid arteries flows into smaller vessels, arterioles, where it oxygenates cells in the brain, scalp and face. After unloading its oxygen, the blood returns through tiny venules into the veins. However, when the shunts open, they create a significant reduction in blood flow to scalp and brain.

At the same time, norepinephrine, released by the fight-or-flight-response, affects receptors on blood vessel walls in the brain and scalp, causing artery constriction. This artery constriction and the shunts seriously deplete blood flow to brain and scalp.

This sets the stage for a rebound effect. In a sudden response to the shortage of oxygen, the blood vessels overdilate. The aura ends and conditions are ready for the migraine to begin.

Common Migraine

During stress-free periods, the adrenals secrete cortisol and other hormones which affect receptors on blood vessel walls, keeping arteries mildly constricted and preventing vasodilation. Output of these hormones wanes during evening hours and at night, and they reach their lowest level at around 3 or 4 A.M. The lower the level of these hormones, the greater the tendency of blood vessels to dilate, making vessels most likely to dilate in late evening or at night. Several hours after these low levels are experienced is the time when most migraines are apt to begin.

Whenever the fight-or-flight response is invoked, the neurotransmitter norepinephrine is released, causing platelets to clump. Platelets are disk-shaped structures in the bloodstream that can coagulate and cause a blood clot. They are also carriers of another neurotransmitter, serotonin. As norepinephrine is released in response to stress, the platelets clump and release serotonin.

Norepinephrine and serotonin are powerful vasoconstrictors but have little else in common. Norepinephrine is an excitatory stimulant that keeps the brain aroused and alert, while serotonin is a natural tranquilizer which functions by inhibiting nerve impulses. Between them, norepinephrine and serotonin work in tandem to control the body's pain process. A deficiency of norepinephrine can cause depression, while a deficiency of serotonin lowers the pain threshold.

THE MECHANICS OF MIGRAINE

Amino acids (proteins) in the foods we eat are the body's only source of norepinephrine and serotonin. The amino acid phenylalanine is the precursor of norepinephrine while tryptophan is the precursor of serotonin. Chronic migraine headache sufferers invariably have a deficiency of one or both.

Immediately the fight-or-flight response is evoked, norepinephrine is released. Swiftly it locks into beta receptors on blood vessels in the head, causing them to constrict powerfully. A few minutes later (typically 4 to 8 minutes), serotonin appears and intensifies the constriction, causing the blood vessels to go into spasm. Artery spasm is further enhanced by the presence of calcium. In vascular headaches, calcium must be present for arteries to constrict.

At this point, the immune system steps in and releases yet another chemical messenger, histamine, which creates inflammation by causing blood vessels to swell.

Both calcium and histamine must be present for the headache process to continue. If either is blocked by intervention, constriction ceases, artery walls return to normal size, and the headache is aborted. Not surprisingly, several anti-headache medications work by blocking one or other of these chemicals.

Next, serotonin teams up with a substance called brady-kinin. Together, they coat the arteries of scalp and brain, making these blood vessels extremely sensitive to pain. Blood flow to cells in the brain and scalp is then reduced.

Faced with this potent array of biochemicals, the stabilizing influence of the body's normal adrenohormone supply is powerless to prevent a rebound effect. In a desperate attempt to bring in more blood and oxygen, the blood vessels rebel with a sudden and explosive dilation.

Cluster Headaches

While emotional stress is often the underlying cause of cluster headaches, Stage 2 occurs without any sensations. Research has yet to uncover all the mechanisms involved in the cluster process. But several experts have suggested that stress hormones released in Stage 1 cause calcium to flow into the muscular walls of blood vessels in the brain and scalp.

The presence of calcium causes blood vessels to go into spasm and constrict. When cerebral blood vessels spasm, the biochemical histamine is released. Studies have shown that levels of histamine are sharply higher at the onset of a cluster headache while levels of other biochemicals, such as serotonin, remain constant.

STAGE 3

This is the dilation phase of the headache process. In all three headache types, actual pain occurs as arteries in the forehead, scalp and brain dilate. Fine nerve filaments (nerve plexuses), which line the walls of these arteries, are extremely sensitive to being stretched. When

the arteries swell and distend, these nerves fairly scream
with pain.

At no time does the brain itself experience pain, for it
contains no sensory nerves. All intracranial sensitivity exists in the membranes, or meninges, that line the inner
wall of the skull.

Tension Headache

Most tension headaches occur as arteries in the forehead, scalp and brain dilate. Other pain signals may be
generated by nerve endings located in the contracted muscles of shoulders, neck and scalp. Several hours after the
headache begins, these muscles begin to relax and cease to
generate further pain signals. But it may be 12 hours
before the headband arteries return to normal size and the
headache dissipates spontaneously. Throughout the tension
headache, blood flow to the head remains constant and
unchanged.

Migraine Headaches

Although observations at headache clinics indicate that
common migraine may be more painful than the classic
variety, from the beginning of Stage 3 on, the headache
process is virtually identical for both migraine types.

Once the cerebral blood vessels dilate, the headache
begins. Occasionally, the pain is mild and bearable; more
often it appears as a throbbing, hammering pain that enve-
lops the eye and nostril on one side of the head.

The pain can become so severe that victims are unable
to walk straight, and may bump into furniture. During
some attacks, the pain is so disabling that the person
becomes incapable of coherent thought. Roughly half of
all migraineurs experience nausea and vomiting. Others
are plagued by diarrhea, dizziness, or bouts of hot flashes

alternated with shivering spells. It is not unusual to see the arteries pulsating on the scalp while veins on the forehead are also visibly swollen.

The pain may reach back and follow the temporal artery up and over the ear and back to the neck on the afflicted side. Rarely does migraine appear on both sides of the head at once. Gradually, what feels like army boots pounding on the skull gives way to a steady ache. The torment can last from three hours to three days.

Yet in most cases, the headache lasts only until the victim falls asleep. When the migraineur wakes up, the headache is gone. The sufferer may feel weak and washed out and may pass copious amounts of pale urine, but permanent physical damage is rare.

Migraine does not usually return until the supply of norepinephrine has been replenished. This normally guarantees freedom from another attack for at least several days.

MIGRAINE TRIGGERS

Whenever conditions conspire—stress mechanisms are simmering and adrenal hormone output is low—migraine can be triggered by a food or environmental stimulant. During evening and early night hours, almost anything with vasodilatory powers can set off neurological mechanisms that dilate blood vessels in the head.

Among the most common vasodilating foods and beverages are aged wines, alcohol, some beers, yogurt, pickles, cheeses, caviar, pickled herring, cured meats, liver, monosodium glutamate, hot dogs, milk, meat, eggs and soy products. Many of these foods contain vasodilators such as nitrites, tyramine or phenylalanine.

Other common migraine triggers include

skipping meals

low blood sugar or hunger

strenuous physical exertion

ice cream or other cold foods or drinks

high altitude

flickering lights or bright, glaring sunlight

hot, dry winds or weather

smog and sulphur dioxide emissions from industrial plants

smoking

pollen and dust

wearing swim goggles or mask

loud noise

oral contraceptives

excitement

abrupt changes of posture

some medications, especially nitroglycerine (a potent vasodilator)

premenstrual period

ICE CREAM AND HANGOVER HEADACHES

Fortunately, most migraineurs are sensitive only to one or two of these triggers. But cold can be a trigger for one migraineur in three. These people experience a sharp pain in the forehead or temple after swallowing ice cream or an iced drink. Often called the "ice cream headache," it is believed to be caused by irritation to nerve endings in the mouth or face. Pain impulses are referred by the trigeminal nerve to the forehead area where they set off blood vessel dilation and create a vascular headache. Exposure to icy winds or to any kind of cold on the face, or to diving into cold water, can also excite nerves that set off a migrainelike pain in the forehead or temple.

Yet another vascular variant is the hangover headache, caused by overindulgence in alcohol, a powerful stimulant that dilates arteries inside the skull so that bending forward increases the pain. In this same class are rebound headaches, due to withdrawal from vasoconstrictors such as caffeine, nicotine or ergotamine.

Cluster Headaches

Clusters are almost always limited to males 20 to 50 years of age. Many have a long history of excessive cigarette smoking and alcohol consumption. A combination of smoking, shallow breathing, a slouching posture, and lack of exercise results in a chronically low level of oxygen intake.

An immediate result of Stage 2 artery constriction is release of the biochemical histamine. The histamine immediately dilates the internal carotid artery. Surrounding this artery is a network of parasympathetic nerves that cause the eye and nose to relax. Pressure from the swollen carotid artery stimulates these nerves. In turn, the nerves dilate arteries in the eye and nose area.

The role of the parasympathetic nervous system is to turn on relaxation. Almost at once, the eye and nose begin to relax. The eyelid droops and the pupil contracts, while the nostril becomes congested on the afflicted side of the face. Meanwhile, blood flow to the face increases and the facial temperature rises. Simultaneously, in a last-ditch effort to restore oxygen levels, blood vessels in the scalp and brain commence a vigorous dilation.

The pain begins without warning and ceases without warning 10 to 30 minutes later. The headache develops around and behind one eye and may radiate to the forehead, temple or nose. The pain is usually on one side only and usually continues to occur on that same side.

THE AGONY OF CLUSTER HEADACHES

The pain is excruciating, boring into the eye and reaching such intensity that the victim becomes nauseated and vomits. On the affected side, the eye becomes red and swollen. The eyelid droops and the pupil contracts. The face becomes flushed and sweat may appear on the forehead. Vision may blur on the affected side. Frequently, the pain is so severe that the victim strides up and down, hand clasped over the painful eye. The pain can be so unbearable that the sufferer bangs his head against a wall or contemplates suicide.

While one headache a day is typical, some sufferers experience as many as three. In the episodic or cyclic type of cluster, the headaches occur only during a bout which typically lasts from two to eight weeks. After that, the headaches go into remission and do not reappear for months or even years. However, chronic clusters continue for a year or more without remission. Any severe one-sided headache involving changes to eyelid or pupil could well be a cluster.

WHO GETS CLUSTERS AND WHEN

The majority of clusters occur at night. Researchers believe that this may be due to a combination of shallow breathing and the daily low point in adrenal hormone output. (Normally, these hormones keep blood vessels from dilating.) These circumstances, which favor dilation, seem to set a regular time for clusters to appear. During a cluster bout, the victim is often awakened at the same time each night by the same blinding pain.

Whenever instability occurs in the balance of norepinephrine and serotonin, which control pain perception, clusters may also appear during the daytime. In fact, during a cluster bout, any food, substance or circumstance that stimulates vasodilation can trigger a cluster.

Clusters usually begin in men between the ages of 10 and 30, often in teenage boys who smoke. No family history connection has been found. Beyond causing a tendency to peptic ulcers, the pain appears to leave no lasting damage. But signs of suffering are often evident. By middle age, many cluster victims have acquired deep furrows in the forehead plus a cleft chin, square jaw and other craggy features, and a coarse, ruddy, wrinkled skin.

Fortunately, cluster headaches are relatively rare. At times, they may be confused with trigeminal neuralgia—tic douloureux. However, tic douloureux strikes in brief, painful jabs seldom lasting more than a few seconds, while clusters last for at least ten minutes.

Breathing pure oxygen is an effective remedy for most clusters at this stage. If oxygen is not available, hyperventilation—taking long, deep, rapid breaths—will often bring sufficient oxygen into the arteries to cause them to constrict and end the pain.

STAGE 4

In all three headache types, pain is actually perceived in the cortex of the brain. Electrochemical impulses generated by tortured nerve endings in swollen head arteries carry the pain signal along neural pathways and through the spinal column into the midbrain and hypothalamus. The more rapid the impulses, the greater the intensity of pain registered in the brain.

In this stage, the pain process is approximately the same in all three headache types.

All Headache Types

Relayed from one nerve cell to the next by neurotransmitters, pain impulses from swollen head arteries travel along the triple-branched trigeminal nerve to the spinal cord. Once in the brain, all pain impulses are borne along by a neurotransmitter called Substance P.

In the dorsal horn of the spinal cord is a neurological "gate." Nerve messages from all over the body converge on this gate before entering the brain. Only a certain number of pain impulses can pass through the gate at one time. When other messages that seem more important are jamming the gate, pain impulses are unable to pass.

Most of us have experienced this phenomenon when we incurred a sports injury. So intent were we on winning or scoring that the pain went unnoticed until the game ended. At this point, messages about the game ceased and pain impulses were able to break through—and we knew we were hurting!

During World War II pain researcher Henry Beecher found that wounded soldiers required far less morphine than civilians with comparable injuries. He concluded that being injured was traumatic for a civilian, and produced great anxiety, while for a soldier, being injured brought relief at being taken out of battle.

Anxiety versus relief work in tandem to control entry of headache impulses through the pain gate. This translates biochemically into pain control by norepinephrine and serotonin, as they also work in tandem. Norepinephrine is produced through stress mechanisms turned on by anxiety and similar fear-based negative emotions. A high level of negative emotions produces a high level of norepinephrine, allowing an excessive number of pain impulses to pass through the gate.

Alternatively, positive emotions calm and relieve the mind so that additional serotonin from the diet can penetrate the blood-brain barrier and reach the brain. A sufficiency of serotonin restricts pain impulses from passing through the gate and also reduces perception to pain.

The Body's Own Natural Narcotics Deaden Pain

From the gate, pain impulses travel on to the midbrain. At work in both locations are two types of opiatelike brain chemicals, the smaller, shorter-acting enkephalins, and the longer-lasting endorphins. Acting like morphine, these substances can deactivate Substance P, stalling and blocking pain impulses.

These painkilling chemicals are also controlled by the delicate balance of norepinephrine and serotonin. A sufficiency of serotonin enhances the ability of endorphins to lock into anti-pain morphine receptors in the brain, thus effectively blocking pain impulses.

While norepinephrine and serotonin are released by the adrenal glands in response to stress, they are also produced in the brain. One way to ensure having sufficient serotonin is to eat enough foods containing tryptophan, serotonin's precursor. (See Technique #5.)

In this way, enkephalins and endorphins effectively control an individual's pain threshold. In chronic headache victims, endorphin levels are invariably low. This is because repeated stress totally consumes the endorphin supply, leaving one defenseless against pain. Abnormally low endorphin levels have also been found in other painful disorders known to develop from chronic stress.

Scientists have thus discovered the mechanism through which negative emotions such as anger, hostility, bitterness, or hopelessness, deplete the body's store of endorphins, seriously reducing a person's ability to tolerate pain.

The good news is that two natural therapies can swiftly replenish the endorphin supply. They are *rhythmic exercise* and *thinking positively*, so that we experience only positive emotions. Endorphin supplies can be boosted significantly by an hour of brisk exercise. As soon as it is released in the brain, endorphin begins to block pain receptors, creating a delicious pain-free high with upbeat feelings of sharpness and alertness. Positive thinking creates a similar upbeat state of pain-free consciousness.

The Limited Benefits of Headache Drugs

Based on a series of double-blind studies at leading university medical centers, approximately one-third of the beneficial effect of drugs comes not from any pharmaceutical action but from the body-mind's own placebo effect. The placebo effect stems from the patient's *belief* in a therapy rather than from the therapy itself.

Through the faith of believing in a medication or therapy, hope is aroused, and the mind begins to work independently of the treatment. It begins to harness the body's own natural healing powers. Among the principal healing forces mobilized by the placebo effect are endorphins and enkephalins. Through a combination of nondrug therapies—positive thinking and rhythmic exercise, for example—endorphin is often released in such amounts that these hormones can completely block severe headache pain.

A dramatic example of the placebo effect is seen when headache sufferers who believe they have a brain tumor are told by a physician that they do not. At least half of these patients show immediate and significant improvement. Their joy and relief releases clouds of endorphin that effectively block every pain receptor in the brain. As they experience this exhilarating feeling of pain-free ease, their mood soars into a euphoric state of high-level wellness. For many, this transformation from helplessness to joy is proof that they can overcome their chronic headaches without drugs.

Those pain impulses that survive the spinal cord gate and the activity of enkephalins and endorphins in the midbrain are relayed on through the hypothalamus and pituitary glands to the cortex, where pain perception actually occurs.

Here again, the extent of pain actually felt is controlled by the balance between norepinephrine and serotonin. Depletion of either can lead to depression. It hardly seems surprising then that chronic headache and depression so frequently occur together.

DEAR DIARY: A POWERFUL HEALING TOOL

Keeping a headache diary is standard practice at headache clinics. By noting the circumstances surrounding each episode, you can often detect the cause of your headaches. Note down such vital facts as the day of the week and the season; duration and frequency of attacks; time of day; and what you ate, drank, thought, did or felt prior to the headache. Are your headaches worsening or improving? Are you taking medications or oral contraceptives?

Was the pain steady or throbbing, confined to only one side of the head? Does it appear singly or in clusters? Does it occur during or after sex, or after caffeine, alcohol or smoking? Was it preceded by a conflict or a stressful situation, or by exercise, or did you have a stressful day at work? How is the headache related to your menstrual period? And so on.

After a few weeks, a pattern should emerge which can help you identify stressful situations, possible migraine triggers and potential vasodilators or vasoconstrictors that could be causing your headaches.

KNOWLEDGE IS POWER

Through acquiring familiarity with each step of the headache process, headaches need no longer appear mysterious or frightening, nor hold any power over us. We now know that by using drugless behavioral medicine we ourselves can intervene successfully on all four headache levels.

Although we've covered all the headache basics in this chapter, you will find still other helpful facts and information in the chapters that follow. Once you have read this book right through, you will be very informed about headaches.

ADDITIONAL FREE HEADACHE INFORMATION

Further information is available from these sources.

National Headache Foundation
5252 North Western Avenue
Chicago, IL 60625
Phone 1-800-523-8858 in Illinois; 1-800-843-2256 in the rest of the United States. Offers educational materials on headaches and list of physician members and clinics. Annual membership was recently $15.

American Association for the Study of Headache
PO Box 5136
San Clemente, CA 92672
Can help you locate a headache clinic.

4 How to Start Feeling Better Right Away

Suppose you're just coming down with a headache. Which Anti-Headache Techniques can you use right away to relieve your pain and to start feeling better?

To begin with, you must be able to identify your headache type and, in some cases, the stage that it is in. That's why we've placed this section this far on in the book. (We assume you have already read Chapters 1, 2 and 3.)

Once you're certain which type of headache you have—*and that it is benign*—you can begin using a variety of Anti-Headache Techniques for temporary relief. These fast-acting techniques are intended only as a stopgap measure to give you time to read this book right through.

To ensure being able to launch a truly holistic approach, the only one that will get rid of your headaches permanently, you must read and absorb this book right through to the end.

Listed below are the best techniques for speedy relief of each headache type. The page number of each technique is given in the table of contents in front of this book. Full instructions for using each technique are thus easily found. The abbreviation AHT in the listings below stands for Anti-Headache Technique.

Cluster Headaches

AHT #8-A: Giving the One-Two Punch to Cluster Headaches.

Migraine Headaches

AHT #7: The Li-Shou Method.
AHT #8: Walk Your Headache Away.
AHT #9: Breathe Away Migraines.
AHT #9-A: Rub Away Headache Pain.
AHT #10: Banish Headaches With This Facial Tone-Up.
AHT #10-A: Morphine For the Mind.
AHT #11: Brush and Massage Your Headache Away.
AHT #12: Temperature Therapy For Speedy Relief.
AHT #12-A: Using Cold to Kill a Headache.

Tension Headaches

AHT #7: The Li-Shou Method.
AHT #8: Walk Your Headache Away.
AHT #9-A: Rub Away Headache Pain.
AHT #10: Banish Headache Pain With This Facial Tone-Up.
AHT #10-A: Morphine for the Mind.
AHT #11: Brush and Massage Your Headache Away.
AHT #12: Temperature Therapy For Speedy Relief.
AHT #12-A: Using Cold to Kill a Headache.
AHT #13: Quick Relief for Tension Headaches.

Hunger or Hypoglycemia Headaches

AHT #3-A: A Proven Remedy for Hypoglycemia Headaches.

Hangover Headaches

AHT #1: Quick Relief for Hangover Headaches.

5 The Nutritional Approach

Myfanwy Jones, a 40-year old secretary in Cardiff, Wales, had suffered from recurring migraine attacks for over ten years. The headaches kept her away from work for several weeks each year.

Finally, she consulted a specialist at London's Charing Cross Hospital. After a thorough examination, the specialist sent Myfanwy home with instructions to completely eliminate from her diet the ten most common foods that experience had shown triggered migraine headaches.

These foods were

all wheat and corn products

chocolate

all whole milk products, especially aged or yellow cheeses

all meats, fish or vegetables that are processed, cured, smoked, aged, marinated, pickled, salted or fermented (including bacon, ham, hot dogs and all types of sausage)

citrus fruits

MSG (monosodium glutamate)

all alcohol, especially red wines

beef, pork and liver

seafood and shellfish

all fried foods and fats

Myfanwy was to replace these foods with any selection of fresh fruits and vegetables, tubers, seeds, and other types of whole grains, augmented occasionally with small helpings of non-fried chicken, turkey or fish.

Although Myfanwy had serious doubts that her headaches were caused by what she ate, she stayed faithfully with her new diet. When three months had gone by without a single migraine, her views began to change.

"I never thought that the same foods I'd been eating since childhood, and that my parents and grandparents had eaten all their lives, could be causing my headaches," she said in an interview.

After the three-months trial period was over, Myfanwy found that she could safely eat wheat, corn and citrus without getting a headache. It was primarily foods of animal origin—that is, foods high in amines—that seemed to trigger her migraines.

Myfanwy's was one of the many similar cases which, a short while later, prompted Dr. Ellen Grant of London's Charing Cross Hospital, to study the effects of various foods on 60 chronic migraine patients. Dr. Grant found that when the ten most common migraine trigger foods were eliminated, 50 of the 60 persons in the study became completely headache-free.

Dr. Grant's is one of several landmark studies made in recent years which indicate that, by changing what, when and how we eat, a sizeable proportion of migraine attacks could be prevented.

GUILTY FOODS

Most clinical ecologists (allergy doctors) believe that migraine may be triggered by addictive cravings for foods that contain amines. Amines are precursors of several neurotransmitters that cause the brain to secrete enkephalin and endorphins, morphine-like narcotic painkillers. Eating amine-rich foods creates a painless high that makes us feel good. We then develop an addiction to these foods. When we stop eating them, we experience withdrawal symptoms. So we give ourselves another fix by eating more of the foods we crave. Regardless of how much we eat, we continue to crave these foods.

The catch is that most foods high in amines are also powerful vasodilators. In conjunction with emotional stress, and when the body's adrenal-hormone supply is at a low point in its daily cycle, amines from foods can easily trigger a Stage 3 dilation and set off migraine in a susceptible person.

Among the most potent vasodilators in common foods are:

tyramine, found in most red wines, cheeses, liver, cured meats and chocolate

octapamine, found in citrus

phenylethylamine, found in chocolate and alcohol

monosodium glutamate, found in Chinese restaurant food and in many canned and processed foods

sodium nitrite (and sodium nitrate), found in many types of cured meats

All foods containing these substances are high on the list of suspected migraine trigger foods.

Some other common migraine trigger foods are:

canned figs

non-white vinegar

yeast products, including
  yeast breads

nuts; dried peas and beans

ice cream

white flour

white sugar

most canned, preserved and
  processed foods

commercial salad dressings

eggs

chocolate milk

syrup

most commercial baked goods,
  especially pies, brownies,
  doughnuts, cookies, cakes
  and candies

☐ Anti-Headache Technique #1: Quick Relief for Hangover Headaches

Alcohol is another powerful vasodilator capable of triggering both migraine and cluster headaches. In people not susceptible to either of these types, it can set off a less severe, but still painful, hangover headache.

Alcoholic beverages which contain esters, aldehydes and phenolic flavonoids, such as red wines, are ranked among those most likely to provoke a headache. If you must drink, vodka is least likely to provoke a headache, followed by white wines, brandy and gin. Another way to prevent an alcohol-induced headache is to eat before drinking and to continue to eat and snack along with your drinks.

When consumed, all forms of alcohol are carried in the bloodstream to the liver where they are broken down into carbon dioxide, fatty acids and carbohydrate. The carbon dioxide sets off vasodilation in arteries inside the skull. This can trigger a cluster or migraine headache in susceptible people. For instance, a recent British study found that red wines precipitated migraines in 9 of 11 patients who suspected they were sensitive to alcohol.

Yet for most of us, overindulgence in alcohol is more likely to provoke a typical hangover headache, a pulsating, vascular type of head pain often accompanied by nausea. It can begin as early as one hour after drinking begins. Some people get hangover headaches after only one or two drinks. Others must indulge in several drinks before provoking a hangover headache. Often, the headache appears on waking up the morning after. Not surprisingly, hangover headaches are most common on Sunday mornings.

Several home remedies will help to relieve hangover headaches. Coffee will constrict dilated arteries and help to ease the headache pain.

But the *very best* remedy is a bowl of strong broth. Failing this, drink a glass of fruit or tomato juice in which you have dissolved a tablespoon of honey.

☐ Anti-Headache Technique #1-A: Prevent Headaches by Avoiding This Food Additive

Anyone prone to migraine should also studiously avoid exposure to MSG, monosodium glutamate. This popular flavor enhancer can also provoke a headache in people *not* prone to migraine. It is liberally used by cooks in Chinese restaurants. If you must eat in these restaurants, try to avoid beginning the meal with wonton soup, a small bowl of which typically contains 2.5 grams of MSG. Endeavor instead to eat some bread first, or any other food free of MSG, so that you do not consume the MSG-laden course on an empty stomach. Another food that may be high in MSG is hydrolized vegetable protein. Many Chinese restaurants will now serve food without MSG if you ask; it's a good idea to do so.

An MSG headache is actually caused by free glutamic acid which stimulates taste receptors on the tongue. The headache begins 20 to 30 minutes after eating MSG and is experienced as an ache or throbbing pain over the temples, in the forehead area, and also in the cheeks and jaw. It is sometimes accompanied by a burning sensation in the chest and upper torso. In non-migraineurs, it usually disappears within an hour.

☐ Anti-Headache Technique #2: How to End Caffeine Rebound Headaches

Caffeine is a legal form of speed that can both constrict and dilate arteries, and can also cause a painful rebound headache. In moderate quantities, say two to three cups a day, coffee is a powerful vasoconstrictor. Yet in larger amounts, such as five or more cups per day, it becomes a potent vasodilator.

In moderate quantities, coffee will relieve certain vascular headaches by constricting already dilated arteries. But in larger amounts, it causes blood vessels to dilate. It can also cause a rebound headache.

A rebound headache occurs when a caffeine addict misses a fix and begins to experience withdrawal symptoms. The dilated arteries will constrict again as soon as another cup of coffee is consumed. And the coffee-withdrawal headache swiftly disappears. Unfortunately, migraine headaches do not respond as readily to coffee, though tension headaches occasionally do.

When suffering from rebound headaches provoked by caffeine, the solution is to gradually reduce intake of not only coffee but of tea, cocoa, cola drinks and any other caffeine-containing beverages or medications. Otherwise, it's best to keep coffee intake down to not more than two or three cups per day. Besides causing headaches, caffeine has been implicated in causing insomnia and restlessness and in heightening risk of heart disease and bladder cancer.

☐ Anti-Headache Technique #3: Finding the Nutritional Fuse That Sets Off Your Headache

Not every migraine attack is triggered by a food. We should never forget that food triggers migraine 1) only when a person is already under emotional stress, and 2) when the stabilizing effect of normal adrenal hormone output is at a low point in its daily cycle. What this means is that without our being aware of it, Stages 1 and 2 in the headache process could have already occurred.

But studies have shown that at least 25 to 30 per cent of migraineurs can benefit from diet and nutritional therapy, while the elimination of trigger foods could probably prevent migraine attacks in as many more. It often is not necessary to give up all of the trigger foods listed in this chapter so far. Only a few may actually be triggering your headaches.

Assuming you are suffering from fairly frequent chronic migraines, you should be able to identify your personal trigger foods by using an elimination diet. This involves a simple three-step process.

• Step 1. Begin an anti-migraine diet, eating only foods unlikely to trigger a headache. If after ten days, your migraines have ceased, this is a good indication that your headaches may be due to one or more trigger foods.

• Step 2. Make a list of those foods or beverages you crave the most and which you suspect could be precipitating your headaches.

• Step 3. Every two days, reintroduce a single suspect food into your diet. During a 48-hour period, eat several helpings, especially in the evening. If you get a headache, eliminate that food and return to your anti-migraine diet for another 4 days. Then introduce the next suspect food. And so on.

At this point, you are cautioned not to begin an elimination diet without your doctor's specific approval. However, provided you do not test more than four foods at one time (over a total of eight days of testing), there is little risk for a healthy person. If at any time while on the elimination diet or while testing foods, you experience any unusual symptoms, pain, digestive disorder or pronounced discomfort, stop the diet and return to your normal eating patterns immediately.

On the other hand, you don't need to give in too easily. Don't give up just because you crave a certain forbidden food, or because it's difficult to adjust to new eating patterns, or because of pressure from relatives or friends.

IMPLEMENTING THE ELIMINATION DIET

Step 1: Adopt an Anti-Migraine Diet.

A diet of anti-migraine foods provides us with the nutritional opposite of migraine trigger foods. Since it is usually foods of animal origin (including eggs and whole milk dairy products) that are high in amines and amino acids, the anti-migraine diet is basically vegetarian. In fact, thousands have ended their chronic migraines for good simply by becoming strict vegetarians.

Not only does animal protein promote migraine but so do the saturated fats found almost exclusively in animal foods. Saturated fats stimulate release of a prostaglandin that causes blood platelets to set off the chain reaction leading to Stage 2 of the headache process. Fats of all kinds also increase absorption of amines.

These facts emerged during a recent study by pain control researchers at Temple University in Philadelphia. They found that a near-vegetarian diet low in fats, animal protein and refined carbohydrates significantly helped reduce or eliminate migraine pain. Seventy-five percent of the diet consisted of complex carbohydrates (fresh fruits, vegetables and whole grains). Excluded from the diet were all fats and oils (especially butter, margarine, lard, saturated fats and shortening); all white flour, sugar and sweeteners; all whole milk dairy products; all nondairy creamers; and all nuts, olives, preserves, jellies, candies or frozen fruit juices with sugar added.

Other studies have revealed that the more a food is processed or preserved, the more likely it is to trigger migraine. It makes sense, therefore, to avoid any prepared or processed foods containing fats, oils, sugar or eggs. In their place, we should eat freshly prepared primary foods (meaning foods exactly as they exist in nature). We should carefully avoid any aged, pickled, fermented, cured, smoked or marinated foods as well as all breakfast cereals that contain anything other than whole grains. Salt should also be minimized because it stimulates the vagus nerve in the stomach through which headache-producing impulses can be relayed.

Among foods which have a history of almost never triggering migraines are

melons	cooked whole grains (except wheat and corn)
brown rice	
rice flour	raw seeds
puffed rice	bran muffins
all sugar-free cooked or dry whole-grain breakfast cereals	tapioca
	homemade vegetable soups
pure fruit juices	mixed vegetable juices
cooked fruits	

Almost all cooked vegetables are safe, especially sweet potatoes and other tubers, asparagus, carrots, eggplant, beets, pumpkin, spinach, squash, broccoli, cauliflower, Brussels sprouts and tomatoes. Many of these are delicious when steamed or baked in a casserole or made into a soup or stew. Also permitted are small, occasional helpings of deep sea fish like cod or haddock, lamb, turkey and chicken without the skin. Bake, broil, steam or boil but do not fry and never serve with any oil, fat or sweetener.

Although most raw fruits and vegetables rank among the healthiest foods, occasional ones have been identified as potential migraine triggers that, in relatively rare cases, may provoke a headache in certain individuals. Unlikely as the possibility is, any raw fruit or vegetables identified as a migraine trigger should be avoided until it can be tested and safely reintroduced into your diet. Among raw fruits and vegetables occasionally identified as migraine triggers are citrus, tomatoes, bananas, avocadoes, plums and prunes; and peanuts, peas, and onions.

The anti-migraine diet should be followed for up to ten days, or for any lesser period sufficient to demonstrate whether or not your headaches are food-related. If your headaches continue as usual, they are very likely not caused by foods and you should return to your normal diet. If your headaches disappear, this is a strong indication that they are triggered by one or more foods you normally eat.

The following two steps gradually introduce back into your diet every food that does not actually cause a headache.

Step 2: Pinpoint the Foods You Crave the Most

Most of us can identify our food addictions by answering these six questions and naming each food we crave.

1. Which foods do you eat most of and most often?
2. Which foods do you eat at almost every meal?
3. When you don't get a certain food, do you experience a let-down feeling?
4. Do you feel uncomfortable if a certain food is not available at each meal?
5. Can you relieve this discomfort by eating a certain food?
6. When you eat this food, do you still feel hungry and crave more of it?

Most people have fewer than a dozen foods which they actually crave. Make a list of these foods in the order in which you crave them most. By way of example, let's say that the foods on your list are: yellow cheeses; ice cream; chocolate; corn and corn products; pickled herring; bacon, ham; hot dogs; liver and beef.

Step 3: Identifying Your Personal Migraine Trigger Foods

Let's assume that after following the anti-migraine diet for up to ten days, your headaches have ceased. At this point, beginning with breakfast, you should begin to test the suspect food at the top of your list; we'll use yellow cheese as an example.

You do this by continuing to eat your anti-migraine diet. But at each meal, reduce your usual serving by about 15 per cent. In its place, add a fairly generous serving of yellow cheese. The later in the day, the larger you can make the helping of suspect food. However, do not eat more of the suspect food than you would in your normal everyday diet. Eating unusually large amounts of a suspect food can unbalance the test.

Test only a single suspect food at a time. And continue the test for a full 48 hours.

Keep a diary of foods eaten and of headache reactions. If the yellow cheese does not set off a headache, begin testing the next food on your list—say ice cream. Test it over the next 48 hours. Start with the food you suspect most and work down the list of suspect foods.

But what if the yellow cheese triggers a headache? In this case, you would stop eating it and return to your regular anti-migraine diet for the next four days. You would then commence to test the next suspect food on your list, ice cream. If after 48 hours, the ice cream did not precipitate a headache, you would return to testing the yellow cheese for a second time. You would test it for the next 48 hours. If the yellow cheese gave you another headache, this would confirm that yellow cheese is very likely a migraine trigger food for you. So you would eliminate it once more and return to testing, one by one, the remaining foods on your list.

Test not more than four foods in any one test period. After testing for a period of eight days, return to your regular anti-migraine diet for a four-day rest period. You may immediately add to your diet each and every food or beverage that has successfully passed your test. After resting for four days, you may then resume testing for another eight days.

If and when a headache occurs, which will often be late in the evening or early the next day, the probability is that it was set off by your most recent test food. If a certain food continually provokes a headache, this is almost certain proof that it is a migraine trigger.

After testing all the suspect foods on your list, you can begin to add back other foods by testing them, one at a time, for a 48-hour period. Eventually, you will have restored to your diet every food and beverage that is safe for you.

There's more good news. After eliminating a proven migraine trigger food for four months, you can reintroduce it into your diet on a rotational basis, that is, *once* every four days. Naturally, if it sets off a headache again, you would eliminate it permanently.

In some cases, chronic tension headaches have also been traced to food addiction. The possibility that headaches other than migraine may be related to food was emphasized by James M. Breneman M.D., when recently chairman of the Allergy Committee of the American College of Allergists. Dr. Breneman suggested that as many as 70 percent of all headaches might be traced to food sensitivities.

Once more, we emphasize that before making any dietary changes, you should consult your physician.

☐ Anti-Headache Technique #3-A: A Proven Remedy for Hypoglycemia Headache

Hypoglycemia, or low blood sugar, is one of the most common and dependable migraine triggers. It can also set off a less severe "hunger" headache in non-migraineurs.

Hypoglycemia can be caused in one of three ways: by skipping meals, especially breakfast; by dieting; and by eating meals high in refined carbohydrates (white flour, sugar and other sweeteners) along with fats and caffeine.

Hypoglycemia headaches frequently appear after sleeping late on weekend mornings and so failing to eat breakfast at the usual time. Skipping meals, or eating junk food on the run, are also common causes. Any foods high in white flour and sugar, or other sweeteners, when washed down with coffee or cola drinks, send blood sugar levels skyrocketing. We feel wonderfully alert and filled with energy.

But not for long!

The body consumes refined foods so swiftly that only an hour or so later, the blood sugar level plummets and we suddenly feel drained and depleted of energy. The low blood sugar causes our muscles to tense and this, in turn, sets off a reactive dilation in blood vessels in the head. Long before our next meal is due, we have a full-blown headache.

Fortunately, in most non-migraineurs, a hunger headache can be ended in a few minutes by drinking a large glass of orange or grapefruit juice. But fruit juice doesn't help once a migraine is triggered.

Luckily, hypoglycemia can be prevented altogether by adopting a simple three-step nutritional program. And whether your headaches are migraine or simple ''hunger'' headaches, both will vanish along with the hypoglycemia.

Here are the rules.

• Step 1. Get up at the same time every day and eat a full-sized breakfast. If you must sleep late on weekends, wake up at your usual breakfast hour, eat a snack, and return to sleep.

• Step 2. Eat all meals evenly spaced out and at usual meal hours. Avoid skipping any meals.

• Step 3. Eat a diet high in complex carbohydrates (meaning high in fiber) and low in fat. Stop all refined carbohydrates and drastically cut down on oils and fats. Instead, switch to fresh fruits and vegetables plus whole grains, seeds, and legumes. You may also have a small, once-daily serving of deep sea fish, or of chicken or turkey without the skin. Non-fat, plain yogurt or very low-fat cottage cheese are other good sources of whole protein.

Breakfast is the best time to eat fish, poultry or low-fat dairy products since animal protein is slow to digest and it helps stabilize blood sugar levels through much of the day. Fats of all kinds should be minimized as lipids can interfere with insulin metabolism, a condition that often leads to low blood sugar.

By contrast, a diet high in fiber stabilizes blood sugar levels and helps the body's insulin to function normally.

Three small surveys of hypoglycemic migraineurs made in Britain each showed that changing to a high-fiber, low-fat diet reduced incidence of migraine attacks by approximately 75 percent, and also diminished headache intensity.

☐ Anti-Headache Technique #4: Vitamin Strategy for Headache Relief

Taken together, vitamin C and a vitamin B-complex supplement are believed to work synergistically to achieve a level of muscle relaxation that has helped some women reduce the frequency and intensity of classic migraine attacks.

Several clinical ecologists have reported finding consistently low levels of B vitamins in chronic migraine sufferers, especially women. Although low levels of vitamins B_1, B_2 and B_5 can each contribute to headache risk, the key nutrient appears to be vitamin B_3, or niacin.

Niacin comes in two forms, niacin, also called nicotinic

acid, and niacinamide. The principal difference is that
niacin causes a skin flush about 15 minutes after taking
while niacinamide usually does not. Both types are freely
available in health food stores in 50-milligram tablets. For
headache therapy, niacinamide is usually recommended.

Although no studies have confirmed niacinamide's effectiveness, the literature contains numerous anecdotal reports in which niacinamide has been used successfully,
both for long-term migraine prevention, and to abort a
classic migraine attack. According to these reports, vitamin therapy seems to be most effective when used by
female migraineurs.

For prevention, you can take 500 mg of vitamin C daily,
together with the manufacturer's recommended dosage of a
B-complex supplement that contains all the principal B
vitamins, including niacin or niacinamide.

Even better results have been obtained by adding two
heaping tablespoons of brewer's yeast to your breakfast
cereal each morning; or by stirring it into a glass of orange
juice. If, in addition, you eat plenty of other whole grain
foods plus fresh fruits and vegetables each day, you should
not need to take supplements of either vitamin C or the B
vitamins. Brewer's yeast is an inexpensive nutrient available in every health food store. It is a rich source of B
vitamins, including niacin. Naturally, if yeast is a migraine
trigger for you, you will prefer to take supplements rather
than brewer's yeast.

Whether you take brewer's yeast or a B-complex supplement daily it will be at least 15 days before the average
migraineur begins replenishing her depleted store of B
vitamins. So take it for several weeks before anticipating
results.

In addition to using vitamins B and C prophylactically,
some women have claimed that by taking a 50 mg tablet of
niacinamide at the first hint of an approaching aura, they

have aborted a classic migraine headache. We have also seen several reports in which women were able to abort classic migraine attacks by taking a regular vitamin B-complex supplement at the first sign of aura symptoms.

Niacinamide appears to work by dilating capillaries in the skin about 15 minutes after taking. This dilation, it has been suggested, could break up a migraine sequence in Stage 2.

Many approved stress formulas include 100 mg of daily niacinamide. At the daily amounts mentioned here, 500 mg for vitamin C and 50 mg for niacinamide, both vitamins are considered entirely safe. However, it is generally considered that no one should take more than 100 mg of niacinamide per day without a doctor's supervision.

If you have any kind of health problem, or are taking any kind of medication, you should see your doctor before taking vitamins or changing your diet. Naturally, should any adverse side effects appear, such as itchy skin, nausea or red patches in the skin, you should immediately discontinue taking niacinamide or other vitamins.

Since B vitamins work more effectively when the entire complex is present, a single B-complex supplement is preferable to taking separate amounts of each B vitamin.

Obviously, vitamin therapy isn't going to stop migraine in everyone. But expensive and toxic drugs are not always successful either. Taking vitamins prophylactically, especially in the form of food, is a low-cost natural therapy available to everyone without risk or inconvenience.

□ Anti-Headache Technique #4-A: A Natural Muscle Relaxant That May Prevent Migraine

After reading the results of two university studies made during the mid-1980s, thousands of women migraine sufferers have diminished their migraine symptoms by taking daily magnesium supplements.

In the first study, at East Tennessee State University, 500 selected women with migraine were each asked to take 100 or 200 mg of magnesium in supplement form daily. For some, relief came within hours. Most felt much better in just a few days. Some women, who had had splitting headaches for two straight weeks, quickly became symptom-free. Overall, seven out of ten women had no migraines for as long as they continued taking the magnesium.

In a similar study reported from Case Western Reserve, headaches stopped in 80 percent of sufferers after they had taken 200 mg of supplemental magnesium for two or three weeks. In another case, a Chicago woman who had suffered migraine attacks several times weekly for over ten years, had had to take increasing amounts of drugs to control her pain. Agony and depression were wrecking her life. Yet after taking 200 mg of supplemental magnesium daily for four weeks, her headaches had almost completely disappeared.

It has been suggested that, through causing the smooth muscles surrounding each artery in the body to relax and dilate, magnesium effectively blocks Stage 2 in the migraine sequence.

Other studies have shown that four out of every five Americans are deficient in magnesium reserves, especially those who drink soda or alcoholic beverages. Many drugs also bind with magnesium and prevent its absorption.

Magnesium supplements in 200 mg tablets are readily available in any health food store. An intake of 200 mg a day is considered riskless by most nutritionists. However, if you have any kidney or other health problems, or are under medical treatment or taking medication, you should consult your physician before taking supplemental magnesium.

Alternatively, you can increase your dietary uptake of magnesium by eating more magnesium-rich foods such as avocados, soybeans, black-eyed peas, almonds, cashews, Brazil nuts and other types of beans and peas.

☐ Anti-Headache Technique #5: Headache Freedom Through Tryptophan Loading

A theory becoming increasingly popular in pain clinics is that foods containing tryptophan may offer a safe and effective nutritional approach to headache relief.

The rationale is that tryptophan, an essential amino acid, is a precursor of serotonin, a neurotransmitter essential to pain control.

Serotonin plays a dual role in the headache process:

• In response to emotional stress, blood platelets coagulate and release serotonin into the bloodstream. This serotonin constricts blood vessels and can readily precipitate Stage 2 in the migraine process.

• Serotonin is also released in the brain where it acts as an effective sedative, painkiller and antidepressant. In tandem with norepinephrine, serotonin limits passage of pain impulses through the brain's "pain gate."

By enhancing enkephalin and endorphin activity, brain serotonin also raises the pain threshold and blocks pain impulses. Serotonin is also a natural tranquilizer that encourages sleep and it helps to relieve mild depression and anxiety.

Availability of serotonin in the brain is largely dependent on dietary sources of tryptophan. In many people, tryptophan has difficulty penetrating the blood-brain barrier, a protective biochemical shield. Tryptophan is prevented from reaching the brain by a flood of competing amino acids, most of which are released from foods of animal origin. People with the lowest levels of brain serotonin are likely to be heavy eaters of meat, poultry, eggs, cheese and other whole milk dairy products.

This may sound contradictory, since these same foods are also rich sources of tryptophan. The problem is that each also contains even higher amounts of other amino acids, all of which compete with tryptophan for transportation through the blood-brain barrier. Additionally, many animal foods contain large amounts of saturated fats, which stimulate release of a prostaglandin that thickens blood and, indirectly, may assist platelets to clot and release serotonin.

Animal experiments by Drs. Wurtman and Fernstrom of M.I.T. a few years ago revealed that a diet high in complex carbohydrates, and low in fats and animal protein, is best for helping tryptophan to reach the brain.

However, except for beans, tryptophan exists only in foods of animal origin. The safest and best of these tryptophan sources is plain, nonfat yogurt, skimmed buttermilk, very low-fat cottage cheese, and nonfat or skim milk. Worthwhile amounts of tryptophan also exist in oily fish such as mackerel, sardines, salmon, haddock, cod and canned tuna. Oily fish of this type also contain EPA (eicosapentaenoic acid) which, unlike saturated fat, actually thins blood and inhibits platelets from clumping and releasing serotonin.

Undoubtedly, the foods just mentioned are the safest sources of dietary tryptophan. Tryptophan also exists in whole-milk-dairy foods, poultry, meat and in non-oily fish.

The most effective way to boost brain tryptophan intake is to eat one or more helpings of the recommended tryptophan-rich foods at dinner. It is not necessary or desirable to eat larger-than-normal helpings.

How Natural Foods Provide Headache Relief

The trick now is to liberate the tryptophan from the protein in these foods and make it accessible to the brain.

You do that by eating a late-night snack consisting solely of complex carbohydrates. Although the actual mechanism by which a vegetarian snack provides tryptophan with priority transportation to the brain remains a mystery, its effectiveness has been amply demonstrated by numerous insomnia researchers.

Serotonin also promotes sleep. And sleep clinics use this same nutritional technique to get tryptophan through the blood-brain barrier of their insomnia patients late in the day.

Either sweet or starchy complex carbohydrates will release tryptophan and speed it to the brain. Among sweet carbohydrates are apples, bananas, dates, pears, raisins or melons. Starchy carbohydrates that work well include beans, corn, oatmeal, parsnips, peas, potatoes, brown rice, sweet potatoes, whole grains (including bread) and winter squash.

For example, dinner might include baked cod with steamed potatoes, corn and brown rice together with a slice of whole grain bread spread with soft avocado and eaten with a small cup of plain nonfat yogurt. For a late night-snack, you might try a sandwich of whole-grain bread spread with avocado, using a banana as filler. The bread should be 100 percent whole-grain and free of oils, fats or sweeteners. Most health food stores carry such breads. Or you could use pita bread made exclusively of whole-grain flour. (Be warned that most "whole-grain" breads on supermarket shelves are made "with" not "exclusively of" whole grains, and the majority are made with fats, oils or sweeteners.)

A Nutrient That May Block Headaches in Stage Four

While it is obviously wisest to obtain as much trypto-phan as possible from the diet, some nutritionists have recommended taking an additional one gram daily in the form of L-tryptophan supplements. Until late 1989, these were available over the counter in most healthfood stores. However, at that time they were linked to a rare blood disorder called eosinophilia. Most L-tryptophan supplements were immediately recalled, and all stocks have since been removed from store shelves. When and if the FDA concludes that they are not the cause of eosinophilia, and are once more considered safe, they may again become available.

Should this occur, you will want to know that L-tryptophan supplements are usually available in 250 or 500 mg tablets. They metabolize rapidly in the bloodstream and can induce drowsiness within 30 minutes. Drowsiness, incidentally, is a good sign that tryptophan has reached the brain and has broken down into serotonin. For this reason, tryptophan nutrition is best carried out just prior to bedtime.

Most nutritionists suggest that, without medical supervision, tryptophan supplements should be limited to a maximum of one gram per day. (However, manufacturer's labels have suggested that up to two grams may be taken.) Naturally, if any adverse side effects occur, dosage should be terminated immediately. In practice, adverse side effects are extremely unlikely but very large doses could possibly cause bladder problems. As pain tolerance increases, most nutritionists recommend reducing intake of supplements and relying, if possible, on dietary sources alone.

Prolonged intake of L-tryptophan may lead to depletion of vitamin B_6. Too, a sufficiency of vitamin B_3 is necessary to maintain tryptophan levels in the brain.

For optimum results, when and if L-tryptophan supplements again become available, it would seem best to combine tryptophan nutrition with daily supplements of vitamins C and the B complex as described earlier in this chapter.

Since it blocks headache pain in Stage 4, tryptophan therapy works equally well for all types of headaches. Best results have been reported with tension and migraine headaches.

☐ Anti-Headache Technique #5-A: How to Avoid Ice Cream Headache

If eating ice cream, or other very cold foods, gives you a headache, it's due to their contact with nerves in the roof of your mouth and in the throat areas.

Here's how to avoid it. Eat the ice cream slowly and in small amounts so that it melts easily in the mouth and does not impact the roof of the mouth or throat with large, icy chunks. It's also a good idea to wait a few minutes and allow the ice cream to warm up to a creamy consistency before eating. Many people also swear it tastes better when warmed a few degrees.

However, some migraineurs have told us that, by holding ice cream in the mouth, they are able to abort a migraine. Apparently, what works for Peter does not always work for Paul.

After reading this far, you have probably noticed an outstanding fact about headache nutrition. It is that a vegetarian, or near-vegetarian, diet almost invariably leads to a steady reduction in headache pain. By practicing the nutritional therapies in this chapter, you may well find that relief from headache lies right in your own kitchen.

6 The Herbal Approach

For years, computer programmer Betty Schreiner of San Antonio, Texas suffered from chronic migraine headaches that kept her indoors for days at a time.

One day at a party, she met a lady from Germany whose hobby was herbal medicine. When Betty told the herbalist about her endless migraines, the German lady advised Betty to take a capsule of feverfew each day as a prophylactic measure. Feverfew, the herbalist explained, is a rather bitter-tasting herb that is conveniently available in taste-free capsule form in health food stores.

The very next day, Betty bought a supply of feverfew capsules and began taking them prophylactically.

"Just as the herbalist lady predicted, my headaches began to disappear," Betty told us later. "After taking a daily capsule for three weeks, my headaches had diminished to almost nothing. I used to just want to curl up and die. But feverfew has become my assurance of headache relief."

☐ Anti-Headache Technique #6: Herbal Relief for Migraine Pain

Feverfew is the only herb to have been scientifically validated as an effective headache remedy. Two studies conducted at the City of London Migraine Clinic in England have suggested that feverfew is effective in reducing severity and frequency of migraine.

In the first study, researchers analyzed questionnaires from 300 migraine sufferers who had been taking feverfew daily for an average period of two and a half years. Since taking feverfew, 30 percent reported complete cessation of all headaches, 70 percent reported that attacks were less frequent and less painful, and 40 percent reported less muscular pain and better sleep. Most respondents were consuming feverfew in its natural leaf form, eating three small leaves or one large leaf daily.

In the second study, 17 people were selected from 270 chronic migraine sufferers, each of whom had been taking feverfew daily in the form of fresh leaves for at least three months.

Eight of the selected patients continued to take freeze-dried feverfew in capsule form while the remaining 9 patients received a placebo. Six months later, patients receiving the placebo were suffering an average of 3.4 migraines per month, and those receiving feverfew only 1.5 per month.

After the study, all 17 patients were given placebos and within a few weeks, all were experiencing an average 3.43 headaches per month. Still later, all returned to taking feverfew and their headache average dropped back to only 1.5 per month.

In reporting the study in the *British Medical Journal* (August 31, 1985), the authors concluded that feverfew taken prophylactically can undoubtedly prevent migraine attack. But, they added, it is not known with certainty that feverfew is safe for long-term use. Nor does feverfew help everyone.

How a Simple Herb Can Stop the Migraine Process

Still another British study made at University Hospital, Nottingham, identified the active ingredients in feverfew as parthenolide and sesquiterpene lactone. These agents apparently block the headache process in Stage 2. First, they inhibit platelet coagulation, which stops secretion of serotonin. This serotonin would otherwise lock into receptors in smooth muscle cells surrounding arteries in the head and cause them to constrict. To make doubly sure this does not happen, the feverfew ingredients also lock on to these receptors, thus preventing access of serotonin. For good measure, the agents also inhibit release of prostaglandin, another essential step in the headache sequence.

Since results of these studies were released, feverfew has become popular with thousands of British migraineurs who normally would have taken aspirin but who were unable to tolerate the gastrointestinal side effects.

A common plant of the chrysanthemum family, feverfew has been used to treat migraine since medieval times. It may also have other benefits. Sixty percent of British migraineurs taking feverfew reported that they felt much more relaxed, experienced less tension, and slept better. Meanwhile, migraineurs who also had rheumatoid arthritis reported diminished arthritic pain.

The Number One Herb For Headache Relief

Feverfew is sold throughout Europe in drug and health food stores in both tablet and capsule forms, and is also becoming available in U.S. health food stores. Because the tablets are bitter and have a camphorlike taste, capsules are the preferred way to take feverfew.

In the London trials, dosage was two 50 mg capsules per day. But many Britons reported that three capsules gave better results. Feverfew capsules in U.S. stores typically contain as much as 340 mg and a single capsule per day is usually recommended on the label.

To be sure that you are taking authentic feverfew, check that the botanical name is *Chrysanthemum parthenium*. Leaves in capsules should be freeze-dried rather than air- or sun-dried.

Fresh feverfew leaves may also be used if available. Like the tablets, they are bitter-tasting and have a camphorlike smell. To mask the disagreeable taste, the yellow-green leaves are usually eaten in a sandwich spread with butter and honey. You can use one large leaf, two medium-sized leaves or three to four small leaves. This constitutes the dosage for one day.

Feverfew leaves are also dried and powdered and sold as a tea. Herbalists recommend steeping half a teaspoon to a teaspoon of this tea in a cup of boiling water and drinking two to three cups daily.

Although side effects with capsules are minor, approximately 18 percent of Britons who took feverfew in leaf form reported allergic reactions in mouth and tongue. In some cases, direct contact with feverfew leaves caused mouth ulcers to appear. They cleared up quickly when feverfew was stopped. Feverfew can also reduce blood pressure, stimulate appetite and cause diarrhea. The City of London Migraine Clinic has advised against its use by pregnant women, though no evidence of any risk has been found.

After taking feverfew over a long period, withdrawal symptoms such as nervousness, insomnia and joint stiffness may appear. Most pharmacists equate feverfew's toxicity to that of coffee. However, the long-term toxicity of fever-few remains unknown.

Herbals For Headaches

While most doctors scorn herbal remedies, they are, according to the World Health Organization, still used as primary treatment for half the world's population. Considering the mediocre record of pharmaceutical drugs, it seems that herbal remedies are often as effective and in some cases more so. Indeed, some contemporary drugs, such as digitalis, are still derived from herbs.

But nowadays, pharmaceutical companies prefer to use chemical analogs so that they can manipulate active ingredients to minimize side effects, as well as to secure patent rights and to lengthen shelf life. Thus mainstream medicine continues to ignore herbs. The FDA regards them as food. And the majority remain unregulated and freely available.

Although herbs are natural, organic alternatives to drugs—with side effects, if any, that are mild by comparison—care is required for self-medication. For example, if one cup of a herb tea per day is beneficial, it doesn't follow that three cups is better. Nor should herbs ever be smoked. As previously stated, the long-term effects of taking most herbs has not been studied.

Nowadays, most larger health food stores have a herbal section with a wide array of herbs and herb teas, both in bulk and packaged. But it is often hard to find herbs in smaller towns.

Herbs for headache relief usually work prophylactically and you may have to take the remedy for several weeks before optimal results appear. Nowadays, too, most herbalists prefer to prescribe a blend of several herbs in order to broaden the treatment. Most herbal remedies for migraine use feverfew as the core but add other herbs like sage or skullcap which are believed to be powerful artery constrictors.

More Healing Herbs to Beat Headache Pain

Other herbs frequently prescribed to augment feverfew are camomile, a nervous system relaxant; ginseng, a nullifier of stress symptoms; hawthorn leaf, which may soothe cerebral arteries; rosemary and lemon balm, believed to prevent nausea; wild yam, said to help menstrual migraines; dandelion root, believed to minimize allergic reactions; and willow bark, a recognized painkiller containing chemicals similar to aspirin. Peppermint, cayenne, fennel, hops, catnip and echinacea are also used as headache remedies.

The most popular way to take herbs is in the form of a tea. Make a fairly strong brew, equivalent to infusing one teabag of black tea in a cup of boiling water. Since some medicinal herbs have a bitter taste, you may add lemon, honey or a pleasant-tasting herb tea to improve the taste.

Packaged herbal mixes are also often available. Since herbs are classed as foods, they cannot bear labels describing them as therapeutic. Yet there is one exception. Herbal remedies distributed by FDA-licensed drug companies are free of this restriction. Currently, packaged herbals are distributed by several/FDA-licensed drug companies, including Nature's Way, McZand and Traditional Herbs. Their products use FDA-approved ingredients and the labels prescribe an FDA-approved safe dose.

Among packaged herbals helpful for headaches are antistress herbal formulas which combine herbs like valerian, skullcap and passion flower with minerals such as magnesium and calcium, and also with amino acids. Designed to relax the nervous system and muscles, these mixes can be useful as prophylactics for chronic tension and migraine headaches.

Among other promising herbal remedies is a tea imported from China consisting of magnolia and petafolia blossom teas. According to studies made in the People's Republic of China, this tea provides dramatic relief for chronic tension headaches.

☐ Anti-Headache Technique #6-A: Help from Homeopathy

Herbs and other naturally occurring substances are also used in treating headaches with homeopathic medicines. As more and more Americans lose confidence in conventional medical care, they are assuming responsibility for their own health and are turning to new and alternative healing options. The most popular alternative to drug therapy is homeopathic medicine.

Homeopathy uses a number of natural medicines. When given in large doses, these medicines tend to produce side effects. The side effects, or symptoms, of all homeopathic medicines have been carefully observed and catalogued over many years. The principle behind homeopathy is to treat a patient's symptoms with a homeopathic medicine that produces the same symptoms. The rationale is that when given in very small doses, a well-chosen medication can cure illnesses that have similar symptoms.

Homeopathic medicines are best prescribed by a homeopathic physician. In determining a patient's symptom profile, a homeopathic physician will consider not only physical but psychological and even spiritual symptoms. Thus homeopathy is clearly holistic. Symptoms are regarded as evidence of the body-mind's attempts to heal itself. The right homeopathic medicine will stimulate those symptoms and speed the healing process.

Natural Medicines May Be Superior

Before dismissing homeopathy as unscientific, we should not forget that the adverse side effects of many pharmaceuticals include symptoms of the very disease that the drugs are prescribed to cure. Certain drugs prescribed for headaches can cause more headaches in some people. Likewise, some drugs and treatments prescribed to cure cancer may actually cause more cancer than they cure.

Unlike modern-day herbalists who tend to prescribe a mix of herbs, homeopathic physicians prescribe a single remedy. That remedy is then given in frugal amounts to match the totality of Whole Person symptoms. For successful homeopathic diagnosis and treatment, you should consult a licensed homeopathic physician. Nonetheless, due to opposition from mainstream medicine, most Americans have been deprived of access to a licensed homeopathic physician. As a result, tens of thousands of Americans, disillusioned with allopathy, are being forced to practice do-it-yourself homeopathy. Nowadays, many health food stores, as well as some drug stores, carry a full range of homeopathic OTC remedies.

To make prescribing easier, a variety of homeopathic health care kits is appearing together with packaged OTC homeopathic medicines. Some of these packaged medicines are combinations of various homeopathic substances. This commercial shotgun approach directly contradicts one of homeopathy's cardinal principles, which is to select a single remedy.

Another important homeopathic principle is that the more times a medicine is diluted, the more potent it becomes. While this also may sound illogical, let's not forget that fewer than 15 percent of all medical treatments have been scientifically validated by controlled studies. And Paul Pearsall, Ph.D. reminds us in his book *Superimmunity*

(Ballantine, 1987) that out of every ten people who see a medical doctor: eight neither get better nor worse as a result of medical intervention; one gets worse—often with the help of a new disease induced by a drug prescribed by the doctor; and only one out of ten (ten percent) actually benefits from medical treatment.

Using Non-Pharmaceutical Medicines

With help from books and from health food store personnel, thousands of Americans are successfully treating themselves with homeopathic medicines and far more than ten percent are actually receiving benefit. One reason is that, used in correct amounts, homeopathic remedies are too weak to cause any harm.

In making your personal symptom profile, use only the strongest and clearest headache symptoms. You must then find a medicine with a match for your symptoms

A homeopathic physician will typically prescribe a dose to be taken about once every two hours. If improvement appears, you stop taking the medicine and do not resume again unless improvement ceases or symptoms become worse. In either case, if there is no improvement after two to three doses, most homeopathic physicians would probably change to another medicine which matches your symptoms as closely as possible.

Among homeopathic medicines most widely prescribed for headache by homeopathic physicians are these (with symptoms as described in standard homeopathic literature):

- *Belladonna* causes headache symptoms that closely resemble those of migraine or cluster headaches, namely a pounding pain that feels better when sitting and worsens on exertion and that may include a hot and flushed face.

- *Bryonia* causes headaches with symptoms that resemble a tension headache. A Bryonia headache is worsened by moving about and often extends from the forehead up and over the scalp and down to the neck. A Bryonia headache often leads to irritability and a preference for being alone.

• *Gelsemium* creates a headache similar to that of classic migraine. It extends from the back of the head over the scalp and down to the forehead. A Gelsemium headache is often worsened by noise, light or motion. The person's eyes droop, and he or she prefers to rest and be alone.

• *Iris* creates a headache very similar to that of periodic classic migraine, complete with visual disturbances, and with pain experienced on one side of the head only. Nausea and vomiting are also common.

• *Nux Vomica* causes a headache similar to that produced by a hangover or by caffeine withdrawal or drugs. The headaches are worst on awakening and gradually improve through the day. Other symptoms include irascibility and irritation. Shaking the head worsens a Nux Vomica headache.

• *Pulsatilla* creates a vascular type of headache similar to that produced by food allergies or by menstrual migraines. It is a pulsating pain, located either in the forehead or in one temple or eye, and it can lead to nausea and vomiting.

• *Spigelia* creates a headache similar to that of a cluster with severe throbbing pain around one eye and deep into the socket. The pain is often on the left side of the head, it worsens with motion, and the head and neck often become stiff. A Spigelia headache often worsens in warm weather and improves in cold weather.

• *Sanguinaria* creates a migraine-style headache that begins at the back of the neck and reaches up over the scalp to the right eye and temple. The stabbing pain is as intense as in a cluster headache and it frequently provokes nausea and vomiting. Sanguinaria is often prescribed for vascular headaches that appear regularly at periodic intervals, such as once a week.

We recommend that you consult an experienced herbalist, or a licensed naturopath or homeopathic physician, before trying to treat yourself. But because herbs and homeopathic medicines are seldom dangerous in moderate amounts, risk of harm is slight.

The important thing is to have already read Chapter 2 and to ensure that your headache really is benign before you try any alternative healing method. Otherwise, herbs or homeopathy could delay you from receiving essential emergency medical treatment.

7 The Physical Approach

Arlene W., a Denver housewife, had suffered for years from the unremitting pain of agonizing tension headaches. That is, until she accompanied her husband on a business trip to Taiwan. On her first day in Taipei, the capital, she was confined to bed with a disabling headache. The hotel doctor turned out to be an older Chinese who spoke English fluently.

"I can give you a modern analgesic that will merely relieve pain," he said. "Or I can show you an ancient Chinese technique through which you can rid yourself of headaches for the rest of your life."

Despite her persistent pain, Arlene opted for the Li-Shou technique.

☐ Anti-Headache Technique #7: The Li-Shou Method

All she had to do, Arlene found, was to stand up with feet about twenty inches apart and rub her hands together until the palms were warm. Then, using her warm palms, she was to lightly stroke her face from brow to chin 30 times in the same direction.

Next, still standing, she was to partially close her eyes, look down at her feet, and continue to hold this stance throughout the exercise. Following this, she was to extend her arms out in front at waist level with fingers touching. Then she was instructed to swing her arms back behind her until her fingers touched, and then to swing her arms out in front again. She was to do 100 of these arm swings. Throughout, she must keep her awareness focused on her toes and not allow her thoughts to wander.

Before the count of 100, Arlene realized that the awful pain in her head had completely disappeared. Since then, for more than a year, she has practiced Li-shou every morning before breakfast—and she has not had a single headache.

Li-Shou, which means "hand swinging" in Chinese, is highly effective because swinging the arms shunts blood away from dilated arteries in the head and into the arms. Simultaneously, the exercise releases endorphins in the brain that also help to relieve pain.

As additional blood is drawn from the head into the hands and arms, the arteries dilate and the hands and arms become warmer. This is the same effect as that achieved through biofeedback. By keeping the awareness on the toes, this condition is then transferred to the feet, which also become warmer.

After practicing Li-Shou for two or three weeks, arteries in both hands and feet remain dilated throughout the day. By redirecting the blood flow away from the head, the Li-Shou method makes further headaches almost impossible.

Li-Shou works well for both tension and migraine headaches, both as a prophylactic and to abort a headache which has already occurred. As a prophylactic, it should be practiced once a day. When stroking the face, avoid touching the eyes. Simply stroke the flat of the face lightly with your palms. Don't rub or press hard on the face. Naturally, if you have any ill effects from the exercise, you should stop at once.

Physical Therapy Can Conquer Most Headaches

As explained in Chapter 1, emotional stress is the underlying cause of most headaches. In a headache-prone person, this psychological stress is swiftly transformed into physical stress mechanisms that affect posture and create tension or spasm in muscles, particularly in those enclosing blood vessels, and in the neck and shoulders. These distortions of body mechanics then set off a muscle-contraction headache, or they may act as a trigger for migraine.

Relief is often as easy as brisk, rhythmic exercise, deep breathing, stretching, brushing or massaging, and using acupressure or at-home heat and cold treatment. Although these physical therapies are completely harmless for most healthy people, you are advised to consult your doctor before beginning any of the physical therapies described in this chapter.

□ Anti-Headache Technique #7-A: A Simple Stretching Technique That Relieves Tension Headache

Developed in the early 1980s by neurologists at Loma Linda University in California, this technique has successfully ended chronic tension headache in 90 percent of sufferers.

The tension technique is simplicity itself. You merely sit upright in a chair and:

1. Turn your head to the left as though looking back over the left shoulder.

2. Place your left index finger on the right cheek with palm and thumb under chin. Very gently, push the head to the left.

3. Simultaneously, place the right hand on top of the head with the middle finger touching the top of the left ear.

4. Very gently, exert pressure with your right hand to pull the head down towards the chest. Just before you feel any discomfort, stop at that point and hold for ten seconds. Then release.

5. Repeat on the right side.

6. Repeat twice more on each side for a total of six neck stretches, three on each side.

Be very gentle. *Do not push or pull hard or force anything.* Simply apply very gentle, steady pressure and do not go beyond the point where discomfort begins. Should you experience any pain or discomfort, or feel dizzy, discontinue the technique.

Neck stretching was developed after neurologists discovered that taut neck muscles are the mechanical cause of most tension headaches. As you exert gentle pressure with your hands, you should feel the taut muscle and fibrous tissue in your neck being stretched and released.

To relieve chronic tension headache, one series of six neck stretches as just described should be done once every two hours during the day. After the headache is relieved, neck stretching can be continued twice a day as a prophylactic measure. The complete technique takes only two minutes to accomplish.

Headache clinics report that most people with chronic tension headaches usually feel much better after only a single week of neck stretching. Within six weeks, approximately half of all sufferers have reported complete freedom from chronic tension headaches. And within three months, all but the most stubborn cases have usually disappeared.

Neck stretching can also provide quick relief from acute tension headache—the occasional tension headaches experienced by millions daily. It has also helped victims of common migraine.

Alternatively, any combination of neck rolls, or moving of the head from side to side, or up and down, or turning from left to right and vice versa, plus shoulder shrugs and shoulder rotations, can benefit tension headaches. However, people with arthritis or stiff necks may prefer to use massage, brushing, or heat or cold treatment.

☐ Anti-Headache Technique #8: Walk Your Headache Away

Whether to abort an existing headache or to prevent future headaches, brisk rhythmic exercise is one of the most successful natural headache therapies. It is equally effective for tension, migraine or cluster headache and it also defuses stress, anxiety and depression. (To abort a cluster see Technique #8-A.)

At least ten studies have demonstrated that half an hour of brisk daily exercise such as walking stimulates the anterior-pituitary gland to secrete beta-endorphin, one of the natural opiates discussed in Chapter 3 that prevents headache pain from being experienced. The studies also found that exercise raises self-esteem, lessens anxiety, relieves depression, improves oxygen uptake and cerebral functioning, and creates an upbeat mood that lasts for 24 hours.

Several of the studies showed that a brisk half-hour walk also suppresses a number of migraine trigger mechanisms. For example, a small study of nine sedentary migraineurs at the University of Wisconsin found that after 15 weeks of walking and running, the group's frequency of headaches had fallen by 50 percent. And if a migraine did occur, its severity was greatly diminished.

Some researchers have concluded that a migraine headache can never reach full intensity in a person who exercises daily. Furthermore, exercise can be used to abort a migraine provided it is begun at the first hint of an approaching headache. Although exercise is a powerful vasodilator, it apparently prevents blood vessels from reaching the excessive stage of dilation which causes migraine and tension headache pain.

To abort either a migraine or tension headache, resist any temptation to lie down. Instead, begin to walk briskly out of doors. If this is not possible, pedal a stationary bicycle (near an open window in mild weather), or swim, or walk briskly up and down stairs. Very often within 20 minutes the headache will have partially or fully disappeared.

Although brisk walking is probably best, any rhythmic exercise will bring additional endorphins flooding into the brain to clear your head. For some people, brisk walking is the only therapy that will completely eliminate a stubborn headache.

You may feel a little groggy after walking off a severe migraine attack. But as a rule, 20 minutes of brisk walking is enough to make the headache itself disappear completely.

To increase the effectiveness of walking therapy, swing the arms vigorously up to shoulder height. This gives a gentle massage to stiff neck and shoulder muscles and relaxes the entire neck area as you walk.

Some headaches are so incapacitating that exercising would be impossible. Even with one of these headsplitters, you will recover faster if you can go outdoors and walk as soon as the pain begins to subside.

A brisk daily walk of half an hour or longer is an excellent prophylactic for all headache types—muscle-contraction, migraine or cluster.

The exercise you choose must be brisk and it must provide an unbroken pattern of rhythmic movement. Walking is ideal because it needs no equipment, is unlikely to cause injury, and requires no prior warm-up or stretching. By contrast, stop-and-go exercises like baseball, doubles tennis, bowling or golf create so little extra oxygen uptake that they cannot be seriously considered for either short- or long-term exercise therapy.

Obviously, if you are not sufficiently fit or in shape to be able to walk briskly for at least half an hour, you should not suddenly begin to walk as a headache therapy. If you are over 35, overweight, smoke or drink alcohol, are unfit or sedentary, or have any disorder or dysfunction that may be worsened by exercise, you should see your doctor before undertaking any form of exercise therapy.

On the other hand, if you enjoy brisk walking or other forms of aerobic exercise, you don't have to stop after half an hour. Long walks of one to two hours or more can be even more beneficial.

☐ Anti-Headache Technique #8-A: Giving the One-Two Punch to Cluster Headache

Cluster headaches occur when arteries in the head overdilate in response to a lack of oxygen in the bloodstream. When pure oxygen is inhaled, the arteries return to normal size in just a few minutes and the headache is aborted.

Since vigorous exercise dramatically boosts oxygen uptake, it follows that any type of active, rhythmic exercise should stop a cluster as effectively as oxygen. And, indeed, this is perfectly correct. Any fairly vigorous exercise, such as jogging, usually stops a cluster headache within a few minutes.

The snag is that many cluster victims tend to be sedentary males who are often heavy smokers and whose breathing ability is already impaired. Instead of exercising, these cluster victims are advised to sit down and do a deep-breathing technique.

Only if you are physically fit and accustomed to vigorous exercise should you attempt to abort a cluster by active exercise. In any event, you should have your doctor's permission before attempting either form of behavioral therapy described below.

• *Deep Breathing Technique.* At the first hint of an impending cluster headache, sit in a chair with your spine straight, and begin a series of long, deep breaths. Breathe steadily and do not hold the breath at any point. Fill the bottom of the lungs first and then fill the top of the lungs by expanding the chest. When you exhale, squeeze the abdominal muscle to expel more air from the bottom of the lungs.

If you begin to feel dizzy, slow the rate of breathing slightly. If dizziness persists, or if you have any other adverse effects, discontinue the technique.

As the long, deep breaths bring a sufficiency of oxygen to the arteries in your head, the blood vessels will return to normal size and the headache will generally disappear. This usually takes only a few minutes.

Although this technique is primarily for those unable to exercise, it can also be used by all cluster victims. However, if the headache intensifies, those able to exercise should begin to do so.

• *Exercising Technique.* Any kind of vigorous exercise that raises the pulse rate to 120 beats per minute for 5–10 minutes will usually stop a cluster dead in its tracks. Exercise can consist of running or jogging, running in place, riding a stationary bicycle, or running up and down stairs. Ordinary walking, which seldom raises the pulse rate above 100 beats per minute, is not usually vigorous enough. However, race walking (heel-and-toe walking) works well.

Since you won't want to stop exercising to take your pulse during a cluster attack, you should undertake a few trial sessions beforehand to determine how vigorously you need to exercise to raise your pulse rate to 120 beats per minute for 5–10 minutes.

Incidentally, no one over 60 should attempt this technique since a heartbeat of 120 may exceed the upper limit considered safe in aerobic training.

For either the breathing or exercise techniques to work, they must be commenced *immediately* a cluster strikes, preferably within a few seconds. When exercising, it's best to stay close to home or the workplace in case the headache intensifies. Naturally, you would stop exercising at once if any adverse effects are perceived.

Cluster victims should also note that a brisk daily walking program, when maintained as a long-term prophylactic measure, can improve oxygen uptake to the point where cluster headaches are very unlikely ever to occur again. For details, see Anti-Headache Technique #8.

☐ Anti-Headache Technique #9: Breathe Away Migraines

If begun at the first hint of an impending aura, bag breathing can squelch classic migraine attacks within 10 to 20 minutes. It has also proved quite effective against common migraine.

This simple technique is based on the principle that carbon dioxide is a blood vessel dilator with the ability to release constricted arteries in Stage 2 of the migraine sequence.

We can easily direct carbon dioxide into the lungs and the bloodstream by breathing into and out of a brown paper bag. The oxygen in the bag is quickly used up and carbon dioxide takes its place.

To accomplish this, you simply squeeze the mouth of a medium-sized brown paper bag into a reasonably round hole shape, place your mouth over it, and start to breathe into and out of the paper bag. Remove your mouth from the bag only when the air becomes too stale to continue breathing. Allow some fresh air to enter your lungs, then continue to breathe into the bag.

Breathe deeply and slowly into the bag. The average migraineur should experience relief within 10 to 20 minutes.

Bag breathing works by releasing the constricted arteries of Stage 2. However, actual headache pain is not felt until the arteries suddenly dilate and Stage 3 begins. To be effective, bag breathing must be practiced during Stage 2; once Stage 3 commences, it's too late. Bag breathing then may *intensify* rather than relieve the headache.

This can be tricky, because no pain is experienced during Stage 2. In classic migraine, aura effects occur for 20 or 30 minutes during Stage 2. *By commencing bag breathing at the first hint of an aura*, the majority of classic migraines can be aborted while still in Stage 2.

Many sufferers from common migraine also learn to recognize the advance warnings of an impending headache. These, too, are often experienced early in Stage 2. If you are very quick, and begin to bag breathe at the very first hint of a common migraine, there's a good chance you can abort this type of headache also. Once the constricted arteries are released back to their normal size, they will not overdilate and the migraine sequence is broken.

Once you feel actual headache pain, bag breathing must

be stopped immediately. Otherwise, it could intensify Stage 3 dilation. And *never* use a plastic bag. Stop immediately if you experience any pain or discomfort. We recommend that you consult your physician before trying bag breathing and that you have him show you exactly how it is done.

These caveats aside, bag breathing has recently become such a popular therapy with classic migraineurs in Britain that thousands now carry a brown paper bag with them wherever they go.

☐ Anti-Headache Technique #9-A: Rub Away Headache Pain

You can literally rub away many headache pains by using self-massage or, even better, by having someone else massage you. Massage works because it increases blood flow to the painful area. It also helps to normalize muscle tone and blood vessel diameter in the afflicted area. Here are several massage techniques known to be effective for relief from tension or migraine headaches.

• *Massaging the Thumbs.* Rub the top joint of one of your thumbs vigorously for exactly 1½ minutes. Then repeat with the other thumb. Continue to alternate back and forth for a total of 12 minutes. Frequently, this is enough to relieve all but the most stubborn tension or migraine headache. If your headache has partially diminished yet still lingers on, continue the massage for another three minutes. Should your thumbs become sore, coat both fingers and thumb with baby oil or hand lotion before rubbing.

Several prominent neurologists have suggested that neural stimulation from the thumbs overloads the brain's pain control gate, preventing headache pain from being perceived in the brain.

• *Massaging the Neck.* Sit at a table. Support your forehead with your right hand, elbow on table. Then massage the muscle at the back of the neck between thumb and forefingers of your left hand. Using a circular motion, squeeze and massage each muscle on each side of your neck. Work slowly up and down the neck. Apply the same treatment to your shoulder muscles. Finally, give the scalp a vigorous rub with your knuckles and then with your fingertips, using a circular motion. Change hands frequently to prevent fatigue.

Alternatively, or in addition, dig the fingers of both hands into the groove at the back of your neck and massage the neck muscles between fingers and thumbs. Work up and down the neck the length of the groove for about three minutes. This relaxes the muscles of the upper neck and relieves the tension that causes muscular-contraction headaches.

• *Press Your Headaches Away.* Headache pain in the temples can often be relieved by pressing the temples with the palms, or with any firm object such as a tightly-folded cold damp washcloth. So effective is this technique that it will often lessen the pain of a cluster headache.

If, during a migraine attack, the veins appear distended on the forehead or can be seen visibly pulsating, try applying similar pressure over the distended vessels. Almost always, the pain will begin to ease.

☐ Anti-Headache Technique #10: Banish Headaches with This Facial Tone-Up

Poor muscle tone in face and head muscles seems to generalize back into the smooth muscles that surround each blood vessel in the head. Poor muscle tone in blood vessels encourages the constriction and dilation that make headaches possible.

Several headache clinics have found that when voluntary muscles in the face and head are toned up, muscles surrounding blood vessels will assume the same improved tone. As a result, incidence of chronic headache is significantly lessened.

Many people with chronic headaches have reported that, used prophylactically twice a day, this technique has diminished the frequency and severity of both tension and migraine headaches. Still other headache sufferers have found that the same technique has brought speedy relief from a tension or migraine headache that has already begun.

Here's all you do. First, tense your entire scalp, forehead and face muscles, hold tightly for six seconds, and release. Repeat nine more times. Make sure that you tense *every* part of your face, forehead and scalp.

Secondly, raise and lower the eyebrows; squeeze the eyes shut tight, then hold them wide open; wrinkle the nose; make faces; yawn; frown; and wiggle the ears and scalp. Continue these movements for 90 seconds.

Practiced twice a day, this set of action steps promises almost certain prevention and relief for any type of chronic tension or migraine headache.

☐ Anti-Headache Technique #10-A: Morphine for the Mind

Acupressure, or shiatsu massage, is an ancient Oriental method of pain relief that can often stop a minor headache in just a few minutes. Given a little longer, it has been known to subdue the most stubbornly resistant tension or migraine headache.

Scientifically, acupressure has been found to excite small nerve fibers in muscles, causing nerve impulses to be transmitted to the spinal cord and midbrain and on to the pituitary and hypothalamus glands. These glands then release endorphin and enkephalin, the neurotransmitters mentioned earlier that work like morphine to block incoming pain impulses in the spinal cord, creating a natural analgesic.

While acupressure won't remove the underlying cause of headache pain, it often provides startling relief. All you do is apply gentle but steady pressure on certain "pressure points" on the body using the balls of the tips of both thumbs, or sometimes the fingers. While applying pressure, you also use thumbs or fingers to provide a rotating massage. Pressure is usually applied for 7 to 15 seconds, then withdrawn. You can return and repeat the massage a few minutes later. And you can give any number of acupressure applications. Frequently, however, two or three applications are all that is required.

Be extremely careful not to use the nails. Women with long nails may be unable to perform acupressure or any other type of massage. Naturally, you can also use acupressure on anyone else.

These are the principal points favored by acupressurists for headache relief.

1. By far the most popular. is the Hoku Point, the fleshy web between forefinger and thumb on each hand. Place the fingers inside the hand with the thumb on the outside of the web. Using the thumb to press and massage, work around the middle part of the web.

Experience has shown that a single 15-second application here can relieve most minor headaches. By repeating every few minutes over a half-hour period, a persistent tension or migraine headache may disappear. Hoku point massage seems most effective in relieving tension headaches or migraines that center in the eye.

Most acupressurists recommend alternate massaging of hoku points in both left and right hands. However, if the pain is focused on the left side of the head, they will usually massage the left hand twice as often as the right. And vice versa.

Hoku point massage isn't one hundred percent effective. But at each application, the pain usually eases until finally it fades completely away.

2. Gently pinch the lower part of each earlobe and maintain a circular massaging motion.

3. Pinch the bridge of the nose between finger and thumb of one hand and massage. Stay far away from the eyes or eye sockets.

4. Bend the wrist of one hand at a right angle. With the thumb of the other hand, press and massage the side of the arm facing you approximately half an inch above the bend of the wrist. Work around and massage this entire area. Repeat on the other wrist.

5. Clasp the hands on top of the head, with fingertips meeting over the crown. Using the thumbs, massage the hollow in back of the neck, at the base of the skull and level with the ears. Press and massage all around this area.

6. Press and massage the temple areas down to the level of the eyes. Stay on the flat, bony side of the face and stay far away from the eyes or eye sockets.

7. For a tension headache, gently press and massage the points at the hinge of the jaw just below the ears on each side.

8. Using the tips of the forefingers, gently massage the hollow area underneath each earlobe. Remember, we said *gently*.

9. Locate the median line running from the crown of the head down to the bridge of the nose. Along this imaginary line, and on each side of the line about one inch parallel to it, are a cluster of headache-relieving acupressure points.

Using three fingers of each hand, begin at the hairline and work up and back towards the crown. Gently press and massage the area along the median line first, applying pressure for only seven seconds at a time. Then move the fingers one inch away from the line. And once again press and massage points all the way from hairline to crown.

From the crown, you can continue to press and massage all along the median line down to the back of the neck. Next, do the same thing along an imaginary line leading from the crown down the scalp to a point in front of the ears. Finally, press and massage along another imaginary line running from earlobe to earlobe around the back of the neck.

Acupressure points on the scalp tend to be about one inch apart.

10. Place the hands on the back of the skull with fingertips touching. Use the thumbs to press and massage points on the outer side of the neck muscles all the way from the base of the skull to the bottom of the neck. Using acupressure on this area often provides fast relief from tension headaches.

11. Massaging the feet to stop a headache sounds like reaching the attic through the basement door. Yet the feet bristle with nerve endings that respond well to acupressure-type massage. When acupressure is used on the feet, it is known as reflexology. In reflexology, however, both thumbs are used together, side by side, to press and maintain a circular massaging motion on one foot at a time.

Nor is pressing and massaging the feet limited to 15-second bouts. One may continue to massage the feet for as long as desired. After massaging one foot, the other foot is usually given the same treatment.

For headache relief, begin by pressing and massaging both sides of each big toe, then massage the fleshy underside of each big toe. Give these areas a thorough working over. If you feel any tender spots, concentrate on these points. They are often the key to headache relief.

Move next to the area between the big and second toes. Migraines often respond to repeated reflexology massage in this area.

Finally, massage the middle toe of each foot, focusing on the tip. If a headache is located on one side, massage this toe on that side twice as much as on the other foot.

☐ Anti-Headache Technique #11: Brush and Massage Your Headache Away

Since biophysicist Harry C. Ehrmantraut, Ph.D. perfected the technique of the brush massage, thousands of headache victims have made the happy discovery that they can brush their headaches away.

All you need is a natural fiber brush with moderately stiff bristles. Rotate the brush in small half-inch circles so that when you brush the scalp, the upper part of the circle goes towards the back of the head.

Begin brushing above one eyebrow and, rotating in small circles, work gradually back around the temple and dip down the side of the face to below the ear. Continue up again in front of the ear, back and over the top of the ear, and on down the neck.

This pattern takes your brush along both the temporal and occipital arteries. Repeat, starting and staying one inch above the previous pattern. Keep repeating and moving an inch higher each time until you finally brush right back over the center and top of the head and down the back of the neck. Then repeat the whole thing on the other side of the head. With practice, the entire process need not take more than 90 seconds.

The circular brushing motion appears to stimulate both muscles and arteries throughout the scalp and neck, improving muscle tone so that blood vessels return swiftly to normal size. Lacking a brush, you may massage with your fingers, using the same circular motion and following the same patterns. However, when using the fingertips, each stroke should be repeated twice.

Should a headache appear, begin the brushing technique immediately for speedy relief. It appears to work equally well for tension and migraine headaches. After brushing, relief may take a few minutes to appear. You can repeat the brushing technique at short intervals. But be careful not to make your scalp sore.

Professor Ehrmantraut has also recommended doing the brushing technique two to three times a day as a prophylactic measure. The most important times to brush are morning and night. Giving yourself a 90-second scalp brushing on awakening is a wonderfully stimulating way to greet the day.

A few tips: the scalp must be dry. Make sure you brush down in front of the ears, and also on the bony protuberances behind the ears. These protuberances are often a key point in the relief of tension headaches.

If you feel a headache approaching when at a social event, or a meeting or at work, it is usually possible to excuse yourself, go to the bathroom, and give yourself a 90-second brush massage. Most types of women's hairstyles will permit all or most of the headache strokes. However, some migraine sufferers have reported that during attacks, their scalp has become so exquisitely sensitive that they have been unable to brush it at all.

It is vitally important to use a moderately stiff natural fiber brush. For more details, we recommend reading Professor Ehrmantraut's book *Headaches, the Drugless Way to Lasting Relief* (Celestial Arts, 1987).

All in all, brushing is probably one of the easiest and most successful natural ways to overcome headaches.

□ Anti-Headache Technique #12: Temperature Therapy for Speedy Relief

Before the discovery of aspirin in 1889, the application of heat or cold ranked among the most effective means of treating headaches. While it does take more time and effort than popping a pill, such modern aids as gel packs, heating pads and hot and cold showers have made temperature therapy even more effective today.

Temperature therapy works on three levels. First, heat is used to dilate arteries during the Stage 2 constriction phase in the headache process, while cold is used to constrict arteries during the Stage 3 dilation phase. Second, heat relaxes tense neck and shoulder muscles that initiate tension headaches. Heat followed by a short period of cold is an even more effective muscle relaxant.

Third, applying heat or cold to any part of the body creates what is known as a counterstimulation effect. For example, if we apply the heat to our hands, our awareness shifts from the headache to the sensation of warmth in the hands. In the process, pain impulses from the headache are short-circuited and we become less sensitive to the headache pain.

Never expose your skin or scalp to any temperature that is obviously too hot or too cold for comfort. If you feel uncomfortable, adjust the temperature immediately. And avoid standing under a shower cold enough to shock or cause shivering. A cool, brisk shower is just as effective. Temperature therapy should be pleasant, comfortable and relaxing at all times.

Elderly people, in particular, are advised to avoid exposure to extremes of temperature. And those with diabetes, or other dysfunctions that distort temperature awareness, should have their physician's approval before using temperature therapy. In fact, unless you are obviously fit, hardy and in perfect health, you should check with your physician before adopting any temperature therapy. Naturally, if you are taking a prescription medication or are under medical treatment for any reason, you should have your doctor's approval before using temperature therapy.

Here, in brief review form, are the most effective ways to use temperature therapy for headache relief.

• *Warming the Scalp.* If you can apply warmth to the scalp at the first hint of an impending migraine, the headache can often be aborted. Even if it materializes, after applying heat, the headache is usually mild and subdued.

Many female migraineurs have discovered the advantages of using a bonnet-type hair dryer. They have been largely displaced by the blower type, but can still be found. And countless millions remain stowed away in attics. If you cannot locate one, ask around among your women friends.

Although bonnet-type hair dryers have been used almost exclusively by women, they work just as well for male migraineurs.

At the first sign of an impending headache, set the dryer to "warm" and sit under it. Some women find the warmth so soothing that they often snooze for as long as half an hour. When they wake up, the headache is gone.

As you have probably guessed, the warm air dilates constricted arteries in the head during Stage 2, and the migraine sequence is broken.

Lacking a hair dryer, you could use a hot towel. Dip a medium-sized towel in hot water at not above 112°F (or at a temperature that will not burn your hands or scalp). Wring it out and wrap it in a single layer of another dry towel. Then arrange it on top of the head so that as much of the scalp as possible is covered. Renew every five minutes to maintain temperature.

If preferred, you could try a heating pad set on "low." But moist heat seems to work better.

After several applications, use your fingers to massage your scalp. Using a rhythmic pattern, work right down to the ears and down the back of the neck.

Whether using a hair dryer or towel, stop immediately if you begin to experience actual headache pain—a signal that the headache has entered Stage 3. It's then too late for any more heat therapy. Heat is beneficial only during Stage 2.

• *Stopping a Tension Headache the Lazy Man's Way.* With your upper garments removed, drape a hot, moist towel over the back of the neck and down over the shoulders, covering the shoulder blades and shoulder muscles. Then recline in a deep armchair. Drop the head forward and place the fingertips of both hands on the back of the neck. Lastly, allow the head to fall loosely back.

Using your fingers, begin to massage the neck muscles on both sides of the spine. Work up and down the entire length of the neck.

In many cases, a few minutes of massage will make even the most painful tension headache disappear. If not, renew the towel and give yourself another massage. Even if you have to repeat it a second time, this technique usually stops the average headache in less time than two aspirin.

• *Shower Away Your Headache Pain.* Another speedy way to relieve a tension headache is this. Stand under a warm-to-hot shower and allow the water to flow down over your neck, shoulders and back for at least five minutes. When you feel completely soothed and relaxed, switch to several minutes of cool-to-brisk water. Try and run the water as cool as possible without provoking shock or discomfort, and do not run it for more than four minutes at most.

This technique should release all the pent-up tension in cramped neck and shoulder muscles. By the time you have towelled yourself dry, your tension headache may have completely disappeared. The method is even more effective if you can massage your neck and shoulder muscles while under the shower—or have someone else massage them for you.

Some migraineurs report using this technique to abort an impending migraine attack. For this to succeed, you must begin to shower at the first hint of an aura, or of an approaching common migraine. Play the warm water on your scalp, forehead and neck. For migraine, it is not necessary to cool off with a brisk cold water shower afterwards. Should migraine headache pain appear while showering, stop at once and towel yourself dry.

• *Warming the Hands and Feet*. Warming the hands and feet by immersing them in very warm water is an effective way to end a migraine attack. It can abort a migraine in Stage 2 or it can squelch a migraine headache that has already begun. In fact, warming the hands and feet with water temporarily accomplishes the same effect as does biofeedback (Technique #15). The difference is that warming the extremities in water is a temporary expedient, while the effects of biofeedback are much longer-lasting.

To get started, you need a small footbath or bucket just large enough to immerse both feet above the ankles. Place the footbath so that, while seated, you can also immerse both hands above the wrists in a washbasin or bucket.

For both hands and feet, most people seem to prefer a water temperature just above 110°F. Keep a hot faucet running slowly so that every five minutes you can swiftly refill both the hand and foot baths to maintain temperature.

As the warm water dilates blood vessels in both hands and feet, blood flow to the extremities will increase. This draws blood away from bloated arteries in the head and into the hands and feet. As a result, pressure on arteries in the head decreases and the arteries gradually return to normal size. Within 15 or 20 minutes, many migraine headaches will have been aborted or greatly diminished.

The warmth also stimulates nerve endings in hands and feet which creates a counterstimulation effect in the brain. According to reports from headache clinics, hand and feet warming works well for at least 50 percent of migraine sufferers.

• *Soaking in a Hot Tub*. For tension headaches only, a long hot soak in a tub bath can work wonders in relaxing taut neck and shoulder muscles. It's even more effective if you can stretch your neck, shoulder and jaw muscles for a few minutes beforehand. Raise, lower and rotate the shoulders; swing the arms backwards, forwards and sideways a few times; rotate and loosen up the neck; and yawn several times. Another good tip is to scent the bath with peppermint oil and also to rub some on your temples. This aromatic has a particularly soothing effect that helps ease taut neck and shoulder muscles. While soaking in the tub, it's also helpful to sip a glass of fruit juice.

After toweling yourself dry, lie down and place a cold, damp washcloth, or a cold gel pack, over the headache area. Within a few minutes, all traces of the average tension headache should have completely disappeared.

• *Help for a Sinus Headache*. Experience has shown that steam and moist heat can soothe and benefit a sinus headache. A steam vaporizer works best. But the next best thing is to sit in a bathroom with a spray of steaming hot water running from the shower.

Meanwhile, dip a towel in hot water (not exceeding 112°F), wring it out and cover it with a single layer of dry towel. Then place it across the top of the face and forehead so that it also covers the painful sinus area behind the nose and cheekbones. Reapply the towel every few minutes to maintain the temperature.

After 20 minutes of this treatment, most sinus headaches may be either greatly subdued, or have disappeared altogether.

□ Anti-Headache Technique #12-A: Using Cold to Kill a Headache

In 1986, a study on ice pack therapy was made at the Diamond Headache Clinic in Chicago. Ninety patients took part, all of whom suffered from acute headaches, including migraine. Half the group used their regular medication for two headaches, after which they used medication plus a cold pack for their next two headaches. The other half used nothing for the first two headaches, and cold packs for their next two headaches.

The overall conclusion was that, when using cold packs, 52 percent of the patients felt an immediate decrease in pain, while 71 percent of all patients and 80 percent of those with migraine felt that cold packs significantly speeded up relief from headache pain. The study showed that while a cold pack is not a panacea, this old-fashioned remedy can still be tremendously helpful for anyone anxious to avoid the side effects of drugs.

Modern gel packs, sold over the counter in virtually every drug store, have replaced the cumbersome ice bag, and have made cold pack treatment available in seconds. Gel packs reduce scalp temperature more rapidly than ice bags and they never melt. However, a plastic bag filled with crushed or broken ice cubes can be used in a pinch.

Cold pack treatment should be used only after headache pain has actually been experienced. It should not be used in Stage 2, that is, during the aura or other warning signs of an impending migraine attack.

Keep your gel packs in the freezer compartment of a refrigerator. To use, cover the gel pack with a single layer of thin washcloth and place over the painful headache area. For migraine, gel packs are particularly effective if placed over large, swollen arteries in the temple. Otherwise, place the gel pack against the forehead.

Most people usually experience pain relief within a few minutes. However, it's best to keep the gel pack in place for at least half-an-hour, by which time the pain should be thoroughly numbed and artery diameter restored to normal.

Naturally, you should sit or lie down while using the pack. A gel pack or ice bag should not be used for longer than 45 minutes at any one time.

Physical therapies are a form of behavioral medicine with important psychological benefits. Using them forces you to take an active role in your own recovery. In turn, this dispels thoughts of helplessness or depression. And your disappearing headaches confirm that taking control of your life and health really does work.

8 The Relaxation Approach

Deep Relaxation is the preliminary step to biofeedback training and to use of creative imagery. Deep relaxation alone has proved enormously successful in relieving and preventing all forms of muscular contraction headaches as well as in aborting classic migraine. Biofeedback is most effective against migraine, and creative imagery is widely used to relieve all forms of headache pain.

Together, relaxation, biofeedback and imagery are the most widely used and successful therapies employed by headache clinics.

DEEP RELAXATION

Almost any type of headache will improve if you can relax. That's because relaxation releases endorphins, the natural narcotics that block pain receptors in the brain and send the pain threshold soaring.

As explained in Chapter 1, the majority of headaches are believed to be caused by emotional stress, particularly by anxiety and depression which trigger the fight-or-flight response, sending the body into an emergency state. It follows that the best way to reduce headache is to stay in the opposite state, one of mental calm and deep physical relaxation.

Practicing deep relaxation with muscle tensing is an important form of behavioral medicine. It requires that you assume an active role in your own recovery and it creates a wonderful feeling of being in control and of being on the path to freedom from medication.

An overall assessment of success rates at a sampling of pain and headache clinics showed recently that relaxation training helped approximately 60 percent of chronic headache sufferers to reduce and control their pain enough so that they could resume a normal life. Most people studied were able to reduce their pain level by 70 percent, though not all achieved total relief. In many people, the regular practice of deep relaxation alone made further pain medication unnecessary. While relaxation does not cure the underlying source of headaches, it is certainly one of the most helpful coping techniques.

Relaxation, biofeedback and pain relief imagery are all akin to self-hypnosis. Among their many benefits is relief of chronic muscle tension. This unnecessary tension not only creates tension headaches but keeps shoulder, neck and jaw muscles tightly constricted, constantly draining energy during much of the day.

Surveys based on a simple muscle-tensing relaxation technique at Columbia Presbyterian Medical Center in New York City found that it provided symptomatic relief for 80 percent of patients suffering from chronic tension headache. Although relaxation appears to benefit tension headaches most, it has also helped relieve the pain of TMJ and combination headaches, and to a lesser extent classic and common migraines.

What Is Relaxation?

During a 1986 study at the Menninger Foundation, researchers Joseph Sargent, M.D. and Patricia Solbach, Ph.D. found that many of their patients were unaware of what it felt like to be deeply relaxed. Only after undergoing relaxation training could they appreciate the difference between tense and relaxed states. One reason is that millions of headache sufferers live in a continual state of emergency and may not have experienced genuine relaxation in many years.

Biofeedback therapists have shown that mind and body are intimately linked. When body muscles are tense, the mind is anxious and disturbed. Conversely, when body muscles are relaxed, the mind also becomes calm and relaxed—a transformation which takes only two or three minutes. And when the mind is relaxed, muscular tension also swiftly drops away.

Important physiological changes occur as we achieve the relaxation response. The breathing rate slows from an average 15–22 breaths per minute to only 4–8 breaths per minute. The pulse rate slows, the mind becomes clear and calm, and every muscle, bone and cell feels completely rejuvenated. We sink into a pleasant state of calm and stillness, liberated from all involvement with anything external.

A caution: because muscle-tensing calls for a brief but strenuous physical effort, anyone suffering from any form of chronic disease, or who is under medical treatment, or who for any other reason should not undertake muscle-tensing, should consult his or her physician before attempting any form of muscle-tension therapy. If you are in this category, you'll want to know that it is possible to skip the physical act of muscle-tensing and still achieve a relatively deep level of relaxation. Muscle-tensing is just faster and more thorough.

Identifying Muscular Tension

To achieve deep relaxation, we must first learn to recognize exactly how tension feels. To do this, lie comfortably on a bed, couch or floor with arms extended slightly from the sides.

Raise your right arm about six inches, make a fist, and tense the entire lower arm from elbow to fist. Tense as tightly as you can and hold it.

Now become aware of the very uncomfortable feeling in your right arm and hand as you hold it under tension. Hold the tension for only six seconds. Then release and gently drop the arm. Note how good it feels as your right arm and hand experience immediate relaxation.

Without waiting, repeat the same tension routine using the left arm. As you hold the left arm tense, compare how it feels with the now-relaxed right arm. Hold your left arm tightly tensed for six seconds. Then release and gently drop it.

No longer should you have any difficulty in identifying muscular tension. Now place your awareness on the face and jaw.

Does your jaw ache with tension? Many tension headache sufferers experience such constant tension in the jaw that it sets up a constant ache in the temples. Constant frowning can also cause a chronic ache in the forehead.

Mentally work over your forehead, eyes, face, jaw and neck, sensing out and identifying tense areas. Most of us can probably identify tension around the eyes. Much of this tension stems from anxiety. But it often becomes so habitual that it continues even after the anxiety has gone.

☐ Anti-Headache Technique #13: Quick Relief for Tension Headaches

A simple tension-relieving technique, originally developed at Columbia Presbyterian Medical Center, may provide swift relief for most tension headaches, and also for some migraines—usually within a few minutes.

Stand erect with feet slightly apart and continue to breathe normally throughout the exercise. Begin by clenching both fists and tensing both arms and hands from the shoulders down. Hold tightly for six seconds. Then release.

Without waiting, tense both legs and feet, including the buttocks. Curl the toes if you can. Hold the tension tightly for six seconds. Then release.

In the same way, tense and release the abdomen muscles . . . the chest muscles . . . and the shoulder and neck muscles. Then screw the face up tightly, press the tongue against the teeth, tense for six seconds, and release.

Now, beginning once more with the arms and ending with the face, repeat the entire process twice more. Finally, do several neck rolls. Shrug the shoulders several times and roll them around. Raise the neck up and push the shoulders down. Then relax. Without holding the breath or stopping at any point, take ten long, deep continuous breaths. Each time you exhale, visualize the pain leaving your head.

If you prefer, you can do the exercise lying down. Although the whole thing usually takes less than three minutes, you can speed it up by tensing every muscle in the body and face at the same time. Hold it for six seconds, then release. Repeat three times before doing the neck rolls and deep breathing.

☐ Anti-Headache Technique #14: Deep Relaxation with Muscle Tensing

More thorough than the previous method, this technique takes you into deeper levels of relaxation from which you can continue straight on into Biofeedback or Creative Imagery. It is an essential preliminary to Techniques #15 and #16.

Choose a quiet room where you will not be disturbed and unplug the phone. Lie down on a comfortable bed, couch or floor rug with a low pillow under the head. Begin by frowning and looking upwards. Hold for six seconds and release.

Press the tongue against the front teeth and squeeze all of the face tightly together. Hold for six seconds and release.

Press the back of the head down on the pillow so that you raise the neck and shoulders off the bed or floor. Hold six seconds and release. Roll the neck loosely from side to side several times.

Tense the neck and shoulder muscles as tightly as possible. Hold six seconds and release. Tense the chest muscles as tightly as you can. Hold six seconds and release.

Raise the right arm six inches off the bed or floor and clench the fist. Tense as tightly as possible from the shoulder down. Hold for six seconds and release. Do the same with the left arm.

Tense the abdomen muscles tightly. Hold for six seconds and release. Tense both buttocks tightly. Hold six seconds and release.

Raise the right leg six inches off bed or floor, curl the toes, and tense the entire leg and foot as tightly as you can. Hold for six seconds, release and lower the leg. Repeat with the left leg.

Next, take five slow, deep breaths, filling the abdomen as well as the upper chest each time. Then resume normal breathing.

Stay relaxed. Place the awareness on the soles of the feet. Silently say to yourself, "My feet feel relaxed. Relaxation is filling my feet. My feet are deeply relaxed. Relaxation is filling my legs. My lower legs are limp and relaxed. Relaxation is filling my thighs. My thighs feel limp and relaxed."

You don't have to repeat these exact words. But give yourself essentially the same suggestions. As you mentally relax each body part, place your awareness on that area and visualize it as limp and relaxed. For example, you might picture your thighs filled with cotton and as limp and relaxed as a piece of tired, old rope.

Continue telling yourself, "My buttocks feel limp and relaxed. My buttocks feel as if they are filled with cotton. My abdomen is limp and relaxed. My shoulders and neck are limp and relaxed. My arms and hands are limp and relaxed. My whole body feels as limp and relaxed as a rag doll."

If you locate any area of tension, mentally relax it before going on.

Now place the awareness on the face as you say, "My forehead feels smooth and relaxed. My scalp is relaxed. My eyes are quiet. My eyes are deeply relaxed. My face is soft and relaxed. My tongue is relaxed. My mouth is relaxed. My jaw is slack."

Be especially watchful for any areas of tension in the eyes, temple or jaw. Repeat these suggestions, as you visualize these areas filled with cotton, until the tension subsides.

Finally, tell yourself, "My entire body and mind are deeply relaxed. I am in a state of deep relaxation."

GOING DEEPER AND DEEPER INTO RELAXATION

By now, your breathing should have slowed and you should be taking slow, relaxed breaths. You can now deepen your relaxation like this.

Picture yourself in a beautiful garden facing a deep, transparent spring. So clear is the water that you can plainly see the white sandy bottom a hundred feet below.

In your imagination, toss a shiny new dime into the

spring. Then, from a distance of about two feet, watch the dime as it darts and rolls and flashes and twists on its slow, silent way to the bottom. Continue to watch the dime closely as it goes down and down, deeper and deeper. After about a minute, it comes to rest on the white sandy bottom. Here in the depths of the spring, far from freeways and telephones, deadlines and pressures, all is completely calm, peaceful, relaxed and still.

Tell yourself once more, "My mind and body are deeply relaxed. I am completely at peace and in harmony with the world. In my mind, I feel only peace, love and joy. I am thoroughly content and completely at ease."

At this point, your mind should feel wonderfully clear and receptive and you should be awake and aware of everything that is going on. Although you may doze off, try to remain awake if possible. Let go of the future and the past, keep your awareness in the here and now, and continue to enjoy every moment.

You can continue to rest and enjoy your deeply relaxed state, or you can continue straight on into Technique #15, Biofeedback, or #16, Creative Imagery. Both are described in the next few pages.

Whenever you wish to return to normal consciousness, remain lying down for a few moments while you open your eyes and move them around, wrinkle and unwrinkle the face, and move each muscle of the body in turn. Then sit up and move around some more. It's best to avoid getting up suddenly.

Making deep relaxation even easier to achieve are a variety of audio relaxation tapes widely advertised in health and New Age magazines. Among the best is *The Relaxation Tape*, recently available for $9 postpaid (possibly higher by now, check before sending any money), from the National Headache Foundation, 5252 North Western Avenue, Chicago IL 60625 (1-800-843-2256, in Illinois 1-800-523-8858).

BIOFEEDBACK

Known in headache clinics by such terms as "Vascular Relaxation through Temperature Biofeedback," this self-regulation technique has shown a high success rate in aborting migraine and in preventing both migraine and tension headaches.

Biofeedback training comes well recommended. Originally developed during the 1960s by Elmer Green, Ph.D. and other pioneers at the Menninger Foundation in Topeka, Kansas, it has since been elaborated on and endorsed by researchers at the Mayo Clinic, Johns Hopkins and just about all of the top university medical schools. Biofeedback training is widely available and its success as a headache treatment and stress-managing technique is unquestioned.

In some situations, professional biofeedback training may be available at quite affordable cost. If it is, by all means take it. Or if your doctor prescribes biofeedback training, you must attend the professional biofeedback clinic that he recommends.

Biofeedback clinics are equipped with supersensitive, state-of-the-art monitoring devices, and with their trained instructors, they can obviously produce swifter results than you can hope to achieve on your own. The snag is that biofeedback training can typically cost from $350 to $1,000 or more for a few sessions of training.

Yet if there is no medical urgency, anyone with some self-motivation and commitment can easily achieve almost equal results with do-it-yourself biofeedback training at home.

Benefits of Biofeedback

A study at Chicago's Diamond Headache Clinic in 1983 reportedly showed that biofeedback helped 70 percent of headache sufferers after other treatments had failed. And a sampling of reports from a variety of headache and pain clinics reveals that after biofeedback training, patients with common migraine have averaged a 75–80 percent reduction in pain, while those with classic migraine achieved a reduction of 85–90 percent. Children as young as eight have been successfully taught to use biofeedback.

Biofeedback works by using your imagination to warm your hands. Tests have revealed that during migraine attacks, hand temperature drops by several degrees. As soon as the attack ends, hand temperature rises again. The temperature drop results from diminished blood supply due to artery constriction. In turn, the constriction is due to a stress mechanism, one of a series involved in the migraine sequence. If hand temperature can be prevented from dropping, the migraine process is unable to continue.

For decades, doctors have regarded hand temperature as an involuntary function over which we have no personal control. But in the 1960s, while studying the benefits of yoga, researchers discovered that we could indeed raise our hand temperature by simply imagining that our hands were heavy and warm.

By making mental pictures, and by giving ourselves silent verbal suggestions, researchers learned that almost anyone can gain voluntary control over hand temperature. That's because the unconscious mind regards all incoming visual and verbal messages as orders to be carried out. A mental picture and a thought are identical, which explains why we must be so careful to think only positive thoughts, and to speak to ourselves only in a positive way. *The unconscious makes sure that we get exactly what we "see" and what we "say."*

Body Talk Counters Pain

As the unconscious receives our mental pictures and verbal suggestions portraying our hands as warm and relaxed, it transforms them into physiological changes in the body. With surprising swiftness, the sympathetic nervous system, which constricts artery muscles, is replaced by the parasympathetic system, which relaxes artery muscles.

Almost immediately, arteries in the hand begin to dilate. As more warm blood flows into the hands, they naturally become warmer and heavier. Even at their first attempt, most people can raise the temperature of their hands by two or three degrees in just a few minutes.

As arteries in the hands dilate, this effect generalizes up the arms and throughout the entire body. The effect is twofold. First, scalp and cranial arteries remain too dilated to enter the Stage 2 constriction phase of the migraine process. Secondly, dilation of blood vessels in the hands and elsewhere draws blood away from the head. This effectively prevents the sudden bloating of arteries with blood should they enter Stage 3 dilation, and the migraine sequence is completely halted.

As we learn to warm the hands and, later on, the feet, we begin to discover that we can gain mastery over our blood pressure, pulse rate, immune system, muscular tension and, indeed, most of the body's other involuntary functions. Thus biofeedback leads to a powerful feeling of self-mastery that quickly extends to other areas of life such as stopping smoking or going on a diet.

So noticeable is this phenomenon that in behavioral medicine it is known as the *enabling effect*. Because all forms of behavioral medicine place responsibility on the patient and involve the patient in playing an active role in recovery, behavioral medicine empowers us to succeed in whatever we do. Compare this with the feeling of helplessness and passivity that invariably accompanies dependency on drug medication.

Do-It-Yourself Monitoring Equipment

Biofeedback clinics have hi-tech equipment that can monitor your pulse rate and blood pressure, muscle tension, skin temperature and brainwave frequency. Seeing these physical functions magnified and displayed on a screen provides a degree of feedback which you cannot hope to match on your own.

Nonetheless, two pieces of monitoring equipment are readily affordable for home use. They are:

1. An electronic digital-readout thermometer that displays the temperature of hands or feet in tenths of a degree.

2. A hand-held GSR (galvanic skin response) device that monitors resistance and displays it as a variable audible tone. Slightly faster than a thermometer, it helps you to learn to relax swiftly.

(We prefer either of these to the adhesive plastic liquid crystal temperature and mood indicators that, though seemingly cheap, have a very short life and a low sensitivity.)

Although not absolutely essential, these inexpensive devices help you recognize the existence of subtle bodily clues by which you can tell whether you are tensed or relaxed. They are often advertised in health or New Age magazines, or can be found in medical equipment stores.

Gradually, as you learn to recognize feedback from your body's signals, these monitoring devices will become. unnecessary.

☐ Anti-Headache Technique #15: Overcoming Headaches with Biofeedback

Biofeedback training begins where deep relaxation ends. So the first step is to use Technique #14. With practice, you can soon attain a state of deep relaxation in two or three minutes. Or, if short of time, you could use the faster Technique #13. Either way, let's assume you are lying comfortably in a quiet place with muscles, pulse, lungs and mind all deeply relaxed and with your mind focused on enjoying the present moment and thinking about nothing in particular.

Now begin to imagine yourself in the most restful and pleasant setting you can think of. Childhood scenes often work well. Many people picture themselves sunbathing on a warm, tropical beach. Assuming you use this popular scene, visualize a few flecks of white cloud dotting the wide blue sky, "feel" a gentle breeze caressing the murmuring surf, and "see" the white sails of half a dozen sailboats dotting the aquamarine sea.

Imagine your hands lying on the sunbaked sands. Feel the texture of the sand and, at the same time, experience in your imagination the warmth flowing into your fingers and palms. Use your imagination to experience all the sights, sounds, feelings and smells that go to create this most relaxing scene. As the gulls wheel and cry overhead, "hear" soothing Hawaiian music and "feel" heaviness creeping over your body.

Focus your awareness on your hands and silently repeat these or similar autogenic phrases: "My hands and arms feel heavy and warm. Warmth is flowing into my hands. My hands feel quite warm. My hands and arms are warm and relaxed. I feel my hands glowing and tingling with warmth. My thoughts are relaxed and I am calm and serene. My hands are relaxed and heavy and warm."

And so on.

Images That Heal

By now, everyone is aware that one brain hemisphere is more receptive to verbal input while the other responds best to visual symbols. Feeding both visual and verbal suggestions to the brain saturates the mind with suggestions that your hands become heavy and warm.

Usually, within a minute or two one or both hands will begin to tingle, a sure sign of blood vessel dilation. As soon as you feel a hint of tingling in one hand, mentally magnify this feeling and transfer it to the other hand.

At first, you may find that only one or two fingers on one hand begin to tingle. Don't get discouraged. This is a sure indication that you have achieved a high state of suggestibility, and that the unconscious is carrying out your suggestions. The blood vessels are beginning to dilate in your hands, allowing more blood to flow in to make your hands warmer and heavier, just as you suggested.

Try to notice which mental pictures and suggestions are most effective in making your hand temperature rise. Many people eventually are able to dispense with the beach scene and they end up by directly visualizing warm, fresh blood flowing down their arms and into their hands. They "see" their blood vessels dilate and they "feel" their hands becoming heavier and warmer.

Others have successfully warmed their hands by visualizing them immersed in a bowl of hot water. Still others prefer to picture themselves washing dishes in a tub of hot, soapy water. Yet others imagine themselves reaching out to warm their hands in front of a fire of glowing coals. Use whichever scenes and suggestions work best to warm your hands.

K.O. Your Headache with Biofeedback

Having a digital thermometer or a GSR device enables you to observe subtle increases in temperature or relaxation far smaller than you could unaided. But even without these devices, the fact that your fingers are beginning to tingle is proof positive that you do have mastery over your body. With continued practice, all normal body functions can eventually be brought under your control.

It usually takes 20 minutes to warm your hands on the first attempt. Avoid trying to force anything to happen. Just stay relaxed and continue making the pictures and suggestions.

With continued practice, you can warm your hands in just three or four minutes. After a few weeks, both deep relaxation and biofeedback techniques can be completed in under five minutes. And eventually, many people reach a point at which they can simply close their eyes and imagine that their hands are hot.

If you feel a migraine approaching, lie or sit down, use Technique #13, and continue right on into biofeedback. To assure that the migraine does not return, you may want to repeat it every 30 minutes for two or three hours. Biofeedback is also surprisingly effective in relieving the pain of a migraine that has already begun. And it will enhance the benefits of deep relaxation in relieving and ending muscular contraction headaches.

As a prophylactic against both tension and migraine headaches, biofeedback should be practiced two or three times daily with a gradual reduction to twice and then to only once each day.

Whenever you're ready to return to normal consciousness, open your eyes and move them around, wrinkle your face, roll your neck, and sit up and move around. Then stand up slowly. Your state of deep relaxation and blood vessel dilation should last for at least several hours. Eventually, this condition should become permanent.

If you prefer, you can continue lying relaxed on the floor and go on without a break into creative imagery.

Melodies For Migraine

At the 1986 meeting of the American Psychological Association, psychologist Janet Lapp, Ph.D., of California State University, Fresno, reported the findings of a study which showed that restful or pleasant music could be successfully substituted for the autogenic phrases used in conventional biofeedback training.

By merely listening to popular tunes or to any kind of pleasant, relaxing music, participants in the study actually had fewer migraine headaches, and they could abort a migraine more swiftly than those who used verbal phrases and suggestions.

Listening to music, combined with deep relaxation and visualizing a pleasant scene, is believed to stimulate release of natural endorphin painkillers in the brain. By using music, there is also less need for monitoring equipment. And music also works well for tension headaches.

In another study at Royal Victoria Hospital, Montreal, classical music worked so well as a painkiller that many terminal cancer patients were able to stop taking analgesic medication. Interestingly, the authors of this study found that the more you enjoy a piece of music, the deeper and more slowly you breathe and the more relaxed you become. A tempo close to your heartbeat rate can be very relaxing. Disturbing music like rock 'n' roll is useless. But soothing New Age music, yogic chants, dreamy Hawaiian songs, or classical or popular tunes seem to work well.

If you're interested in taking some of the best biofeedback training available, write: The Menninger Clinic, Box 829, Topeka KS 66601.

CREATIVE IMAGERY

Thirty-two-year-old Jim Bell of West Palm Beach, Florida, had suffered for years from agonizing tension headaches. Only constant medication could deaden the pain. But at the local Wickershaw Counseling Clinic, therapists taught Jim to use his imagination to relieve his pain.

Whenever a headache strikes, Jim lies down and goes into a state of deep relaxation. Then he asks himself what his headache pain feels like. His answer is the first thought that enters his mind.

"My headache feels like a knife plunged through my temple," he may tell himself.

"What would soothe this pain?" he asks himself.

"A block of ice," his mind may reply.

Jim then visualizes a knife plunged deep into his aching temple. On his inner video screen, he "sees" and "feels" the knife being slowly withdrawn from the painful area. As soon as it is withdrawn, he "sees" the upper part of his head encased in a block of ice.

"These images always stop the pain within a few minutes," Jim reports. "The painful area in my head becomes numb. And in fifteen minutes, the headache is completely gone."

Jim is one of thousands of former chronic headache sufferers whose pain has been relieved by a visualization process known as Creative Imagery.

C. Norman Shealy M.D., founder of the Pain and Health Rehabilitation Center, La Crosse, Wisconsin, has stated that he found relaxation and visualization techniques to be the single most important therapy pain clinics can offer to chronically ill individuals with a wide range of problems.

Mind as a Healing Tool

Creative imagery consists of making mental pictures and reinforcing them with silent but strongly positive autogenic phrases or suggestions. By using visual symbols plus verbal affirmations, we create an inner dialog that is immediately understood by both the verbally oriented left brain and the visually oriented right brain.

Our symbols and suggestions are fed through these twin brain hemispheres into the subconscious. Since the subconscious uncritically accepts all symbols and suggestions fed into it, our instructions are immediately relayed to the autonomic nervous system (ANS) to be carried out.

ANS pathways parallel all arterial blood vessels and they control blood vessel diameter. They also control all involuntary body functions from blood pressure to heartbeat and breathing rates, kidney function, immunocompetence, digestion, and production of enzymes and hormones.

By learning to speak the language of the right brain—using symbols and imagery instead of words—our blueprint for wellness is communicated directly through the ANS to the involuntary controls of most bodily functions. And whatever we have visualized and suggested gradually becomes a reality.

Once you have learned deep relaxation, creative imagery is easy to learn and results often come swiftly. At the UCLA Medical School, headache pain was relieved in 60 percent of sufferers the first time they used creative imagery.

Nor do we have to tell the body what to do to relieve headache pain. All we need do is visualize ourselves free of headache, in perfect health, and able to do everything that headaches normally prevent. You don't need to tell the mind how to achieve headache freedom. The subconscious will figure that out at the subclinical level.

Therapeutic Imagery Works Wonders

All you need do is make clear, vivid images and, if possible, "feel," "smell," "hear," and "experience" these images in your mind.

If you do know what actions your body should take, it's fine to visualize this happening. For example, you might visualize the arteries in your head dilating during Stage 2, or constricting during Stage 3. If you aren't sure exactly what arteries look like, symbols are equally effective. You can visualize arteries as a rubber hose, and smooth muscles as fingers clamping down on the hose and restricting the blood flow through it.

Although several popular visualizations are given later, no standard programming exists for creative imagery. You can simply make up your own visualizations and reinforce them with autogenic phrases that best fit the particular headache symptoms you wish to alleviate.

Avoid phrases that use the future tense, such as "My headache will have disappeared by next week." Instead, use the present tense and phrase all suggestions as though your headache had already disappeared.

For example, "The pain in my eye (or temple) has already disappeared. As the ice numbs my headache pain, I feel perfectly comfortable and free of pain. Every vestige of headache pain has already disappeared. I feel very comfortable and at ease."

All phrases must be strongly positive. Avoid negatives such as "I will not," or "don't" or "I won't" or "I will try to." Employ only strong, active, positive phrases and talk as though your headache or other symptoms had already vanished.

Turn On Your Own Placebo Effect

We cannot overemphasize here that your success depends on visualizing yourself as *already free* of headache pain. Pictures and phrases such as "My headache will disappear," make weak, vague instructions to feed to the subconscious. Compare it with "My headache is gone. I am completely free of headache pain."

In a sense, we are mobilizing our own placebo effect. And the key to turning on this self-healing power is a strong belief and implicit trust in the body's own ability to heal itself—a force that we can most easily harness through creative imagery.

For proof, a recent survey of cases of spontaneous remission from terminal cancer found that, without a single exception, every person had possessed a powerful and unswerving belief in his or her ability to recover completely.

We can help reinforce this belief by ending our imagery session with an expression of gratitude for having been healed—even though the healing may not have yet occurred. The vital thing is to "see" ourselves as already healed. Try to feel deeply grateful as you repeat phrases such as, "I am happy and delighted to be free of headache pain. I feel comfort, health and happiness all over my body."

Wind up your imagery session by making strong pictures of yourself already free of headaches and completely recovered. See yourself bicycling through Europe, playing tennis, cross-country skiing or doing whatever it is that your headaches may have prevented.

☐ Anti-Headache Technique #16: Extinguish Pain with Creative Imagery

The first step in creative imagery is to enter deep relaxation (Technique #14). Although not essential, you can deepen this relaxation by adding biofeedback (Technique #15).

You should now be lying down, deeply relaxed. Begin by getting in touch with your headache pain and experiencing it. Exactly where is it? What are its dimensions? Is it constant or pulsating? Can you give it a shape, color, smell or taste?

Then continue with one or more of these frequently-used imagery techniques.

• *Project Your Headache Out of the Body.* Place your awareness on the location of the headache. Visualize its exact shape and dimensions. Now detach this block of pain out of your head and see it several feet in front of you. Meanwhile, visualize a gaping empty space in your head where the pain was formerly located. For instance, you might picture your entire forehead removed from your body.

You can do several things with the painful area you have just detached. You might "see" yourself dropping it into a garbage can. Connect the can to a hot-air balloon and watch it soar away out of sight, never to be seen again.

Or you can visualize the detached painful area out in front of you and fill it with ice-cold water. After it is completely numbed and blue with cold, return it to your head.

Or you can magnify the detached painful area to ten times its original size. Then shrink it down to one-tenth its original size. Repeat this exercise ten times. When back to normal size, fill the painful area with a soothing, bright green light. After a few minutes, return it to your head.

Usually, these exercises so overload the brain with sensory stimulation that pain impulses have difficulty getting through. By the time the exercises are over, the headache has often disappeared.

• *Switch Off the Pain.* Visualize the nerve fiber leading from the painful area in your head to the pain gate in your brain and on to the pain receptors. Just before the fiber enters the pain gate, visualize a large switch operated by an equally large lever. As you experience the headache pain, see yourself pulling down the lever. With a loud clang, you turn off the switch. In many cases, the pain suddenly ends.

As this is a brief visualization, repeat it several times. Eventually, the ANS will turn off the pain gate switch just as you visualized.

• *Displace the Pain.* Focus your awareness on the painful area and briefly experience the pain. Then transfer your awareness, together with the pain, to any other area of your body such as your left foot or right hand. You should feel the pain in this new location, often quite intensely. Meanwhile, the headache area becomes increasingly pain-free.

Repeat several times until almost all of the pain is in the new location. Finally, visualize the pain leaving the new location by flowing out into the air. By this time, the original headache site should be virtually pain-free.

A variation on this is to imagine the headache pain diffused and spread out equally all over the body.

• *Glove Anesthesia.* Visualize one of your hands immersed in an imaginary bucket of hot water. As you maintain this picture, your hand should become quite warm. As soon as you feel this warmth, visualize your other hand plunged into an imaginary bucket of cold water filled with slush ice. In a short time, your hand will feel numbed with cold and it will tingle as if asleep.

Now use this phrase: "I now transfer this numbness to the headache area by touching it with my cold hand." As you repeat this autogenic phrase, place your cold hand against the headache area. Almost everyone experiences a cold, pain-numbing feeling in the head while the headache diminishes.

Repeated several times, this imagery often produces quite dramatic results, even when medication has failed. It is especially effective for migraine relief.

• *Distorting Time.* The rationale behind this popular hypnotic therapy is that time seems to drag endlessly during periods of discomfort while it literally flies during a pleasant experience.

Picture yourself experiencing the most pleasurable sensations you can think of—being given a massage in a luxurious room while beautiful girls bring food and drink—or whatever else arouses sensations of hedonism and deep pleasure. Continue to daydream as you visualize a series of rich pleasures.

As you enjoy the mental feeling, time will begin to fly past just as if you had actually experienced the pleasures you fantasized. And as the passage of time is reversed, so you will find, is your headache pain.

• *Bathing the Painful Area in Sunshine.* Picture a bright ray of healing sunshine flooding the headache area. As you hold this mental picture, repeat autogenic phrases such as these: "My head is entirely free of pain. I feel happy, relaxed and comfortable all over. As the sun's healing rays enter my head, I am completely free of pain. I feel deeply grateful that my inner healing power has restored me to pain-free health."

A few minutes of this imagery usually cuts most headache pain in half. And a few more minutes often ends it completely.

Other Ways to Harness Your Inner Healing Power

Don't forget the technique used by Jim Bell in the opening paragraphs of this section. When using this technique, you can also see your pain as a row of nails driven into your scalp; or you could see your neck muscles tied into knots; or you might visualize your head on fire. As you draw out the nails, untie the neck muscles or extinguish the fire with cold water, your headache diminishes and disappears.

The variety of healing visualizations you can invent is almost endless. You can create images and suggestions to reinforce the effects of any other technique in this book, or to boost the effects of medication or medical treatment.

Creative imagery won't replace such needed therapies as exercise or nutrition, but it can work wonders in reinforcing their benefits. We should also realize that imagery is not a substitute for needed medical treatment. It should not be used to mask pain that has not been medically diagnosed and declared benign.

For best results, you should practice creative imagery three times a day for about fifteen minutes each time. Some people have experienced swift results. In others, it may take several weeks, or possibly longer, for the necessary physiological changes to take place. As new neural pathways and improved behaviors occur, you can gradually reduce the number of daily sessions.

Write Your Headaches Away

Suppose you have trouble making mental images? If so, try writing down your autogenic phrases and suggestions. Enter deep relaxation as usual. Then get up and sit at a table and write down your suggestions. Write them over and over. Writing automatically creates strong mental images of the very suggestions you are writing. Even people with superior imaging ability have obtained still better results by writing.

Since you may get what you "see," it is best not to involve the eyes or other fragile organs in any kind of psycho-technique. Avoid "removing" the eyes from the head or driving an imaginary nail or knife into the eyes. Use an alternative visualization instead.

Imagery techniques should not be used by anyone with any kind of mental instability or mental illness, or who is subject to hallucinations or who, for any other reason, might be adversely affected by using imagery and visualizations. We recommend seeing your doctor before practicing creative imagery.

9 The Positive Approach

Only in recent years have some headache clinics begun to confront the root cause of all headaches, and to stop headaches where they begin, namely in our belief systems. Most appropriately called *cognitive positivism,* this powerful form of behavioral medicine emerged from recent discoveries in immunity research. It was found that the largest single influence on our health and well-being consists of our emotions.

When our emotions are positive, we are able to enter a state of relaxation. We feel calm and relaxed and terrific all over. Our immunity soars and we swiftly become twice as resistant to cancer and all infections. Our arteries relax, our blood pressure drops, and we become virtually immune to heart disease, diabetes, kidney disease and all the other chronic diseases that kill and plague Americans. At the same time, we become almost equally immune to all types of headaches.

When our emotions are negative, we enter the opposite state. We become prone to cancer and infections, our blood pressure rises, and we become increasingly at risk for every type of disease and dysfunction. At the same time, our susceptibility to all types of headaches begins to soar.

The actual process by which inappropriate conditioned beliefs are translated into physiological diseases and into headaches is described in detail under the heading ''Stage One'' in Chapter 3. This section concludes with the advice that we drop all beliefs that intensify headache pain and replace them with new beliefs that minimize headache pain or that can actually liberate us from headaches altogether.

□ Anti-Headache Technique #17: Liberate Yourself from Headaches with Cognitive Positivism

Let us begin by restating the psychological axiom that every feeling is triggered in the context of a preceding thought . . . and that each thought that arises is determined by the context of the beliefs that we hold.

Every negative feeling is preceded by a negative thought that arises from holding one or more negative beliefs. Likewise, every positive feeling is preceded by a positive thought that arises from holding one or more positive beliefs.

It doesn't take a genius to figure out that if we drop our negative beliefs and replace them with positive beliefs, we are not only going to have a shot at feeling good all the time, but also that we can become virtually free of headaches and minimize our risk of getting almost any other disease or dysfunction. By changing our beliefs, we change the way we perceive potentially stressful life events.

For example, Smith and Jones are both laid off from their production-line jobs in an outdated plant. Smith fears that he will be unable to find another job. The thought of losing his home, furniture and car, and of being unable to support his family, makes him increasingly anxious and depressed. As Smith continues to perceive the situation in a fearful way, his anxiety increases and he begins to experience frequent tension headaches.

Jones, by contrast, perceives his job loss as a fortunate release from a boring occupation and as a wonderful opportunity to train for a new career in computers. Rather than getting headaches, Jones feels totally confident and capable, an upbeat mindset boosted by secretion of endorphins resulting from his positive feelings.

Although fictional, this illustration is repeated in real life millions of times each day. Both Smith and Jones perceived the same potentially stressful life event. But while Smith perceived unemployment in a negative way that created stress and headaches, Jones perceived his job loss as an opportunity for advancement—a positive viewpoint that left him completely free of both stress and headaches.

When we program the biocomputer that we call the brain with negative beliefs, we get out negative feelings and headaches. When we program it with positive beliefs, we get out positive feelings and freedom from headaches.

If that sounds oversimplified, it's because we are dealing only with cause and effect. The actual bodymind mechanisms involved in the computer analogy are extremely complex. Yet in behavioral medicine, it isn't essential to know *how* the mind or body works—results are what count. And the results we want are the results Jones got.

The big question is: How could Smith change his beliefs so that he too could perceive unemployment in the same stress-free way as Jones?

Healing with the Mind

A key element of the answer is a basic principle of modern psychology—that there are only two root emotions, fear and love. All fear-based feelings are negative, and they include anger, hostility, guilt, resentment, bitterness, frustration, envy, dissatisfaction, anxiety, helplessness, hopelessness and depression. All love-based feelings are positive, and they include joy, peace, generosity, forgiveness, compassion and contentment.

Applying this to Smith and Jones, we see that by viewing life through a filter of fear-based beliefs, Smith perceived a hostile, unfriendly and threatening world. Such a negative way of looking at things intensifies all forms of headache and all types of dysfunctions.

By contrast, Jones viewed life through a filter of love-based beliefs, as a result of which he perceived a friendly, loving and nonthreatening world. Consequently, he remained free of headaches and disease, he felt great, and he continued to enjoy a high level of wellness.

We Can Feel Any Way We Want to Feel

Psychologists have also learned that we can feel any way we want to feel at any time by placing an appropriate thought in our mind. Should a negative thought intrude on our inner video screen, we can easily slide it off. And we can then replace it with a positive visualization, such as a tropical beach scene, before the negative thought has had time to trigger a headache-producing emotion.

In contrast, once a negative emotion has pervaded our consciousness, the strong feelings and upset that it causes can rule us for hours, preventing rational thought and causing us to lash out at people with whom we have close relationships. The result is that we often end up with a tension or migraine headache.

Thinking a thought, incidentally, is the same as creating a mental image, or making a mental picture, or visualizing something. Each of us has complete personal control over our thoughts. For example, close your eyes and visualize a red rose; then picture a snow-capped mountain peak; then a dog.

Were you able to see these objects in your mind's eye? Great! Then this proves that you have the ability to replace thoughts about a rose with alternative thoughts about mountains or dogs. And so it is with negative thoughts that provoke headaches. We can easily slide any negative thought out of our mind and replace it with a more positive thought.

While thoughts can be changed in a split second, it is much more difficult to change a negative feeling.

Think a thought or make a mental picture or visualize an image of a friend or neighbor who has a more exciting spouse, a larger house, a more prestigious job, and a more luxurious car than you do, and you've set yourself up for strong feelings of envy and possibly resentment. Within a few minutes, these negative feelings will start low-level stress mechanisms simmering and you will begin to feel tense, uncomfortable and upset.

Thoughts That Heal

It's not easy to change a strong negative feeling like that once it has begun. But it would have been extremely easy to slide that first thought off your mind when you began comparing yourself with someone else and to replace it with a scene of a beautiful beach. In the process, you could have prevented the unpleasant feeling of envy and continued to feel calm and relaxed.

We must never forget that, at any time, we can personally choose to feel any way we want to feel by placing an appropriate thought on our inner movie screen. Granted, we may have to slide an unwanted thought out of our mind half a dozen times in a row. But by doing so, the mind soon gets the message that negative thoughts are unwelcome. Within a short while, we will find ourselves free of the unwanted thought. And we will also find ourselves free of the headache that the unwanted thought might have triggered.

Learning to control our thoughts isn't really as difficult as most of us believe. Researchers at the University of Pennsylvania and other university medical schools have completely reversed tens of thousands of cases of severe depression by teaching patients to think positively. Called *cognitive therapy*, this method is based on the discovery that many cases of depression are caused not by some complex biological process deep within the body or by the subconscious mind, but by ten easily-recognizable ways in which we distort our thinking by using a negative approach.

Take Charge of Your Headache With Cognitive Positivism

When cognitive therapy is teamed up with positivism, we get *cognitive positivism*, the most powerful healing tool in the entire field of behavioral medicine.

Positivism is simply the opposite of negativity. It implies that we hold only positive beliefs, thoughts and emotions. When we do, we perceive the world in a friendly, nonthreatening way and our minds become calm and relaxed. Swiftly, the hypothalamus recognizes this calm mindset and turns on the Relaxation Response. The entire mind-body enters a calm, relaxed and healthful state in which it remains for as long as we continue to hold a positive mindset.

For as long as we remain in the Relaxation Response, we have no downers or bad moments or bad days and we continue to enjoy every moment of every day. As a result, we experience unbroken high-level wellness and we remain completely free of headaches and other diseases or dysfunctions.

"But I couldn't possibly live like that," you might say. "I need to get angry so I can appreciate the calm periods in between. And how could I feel happy unless I have blue periods to contrast them with?"

If that or something like it was your response, you have probably diagnosed the cause of your headaches.

In reality, the only time we need to experience a fear-based emotion is when we are actually threatened by physical danger. Other "reasons" are all too often excuses by people who prefer the stimulation of strong emotions to the seemingly unexciting alternative of experiencing unbroken calm, joy and inner peace.

There are two easy ways to recognize when we are being run by fear-based beliefs. One is that we may feel too tense and upset to experience calm and relaxation or to use sound, rational, unbiased judgment. Another is that we are coming from a position of scarcity and lack.

When our awareness is guided by fear-based beliefs, we are concerned only with *getting* our own self-interests satisfied. This translates into *getting* security; *getting* enough sex, food and stimulation; and *getting* power through being right or claiming territory or manipulating people; or *getting* more possessions, prestige, fame, recognition, or achievements. On this low level of consciousness—which is where most people spend most of their time—we are primarily concerned with *getting* rather than with giving.

All these positions are based on fear: the fear that there won't be enough to go around; that we won't get our fair share; that our rights may be violated; or that we won't be accorded recognition or prestige. While beliefs on this low level may appear to bring us temporary pleasure, they almost never lead to lasting happiness or satisfaction. All too often they are the cause of chronic headaches.

Worn-Out Beliefs

The headache-causing beliefs we need to let go of are known in psychology as *conditioned* beliefs. Many were picked up in early childhood or in school or in the armed forces or were learned from parents, teachers and other people. Some may have been appropriate in past situations, but the majority are inappropriate to our present lifestyle and they are filling our lives with emotional stress.

These conditioned beliefs based on the past cause us to perceive events in our present lives as stressful. The ultimate way to eliminate the stress that is causing our headaches is to change the way we perceive life events so that we now see them as nonthreatening.

We do that by restructuring our belief system, by letting go of the fear-based beliefs that cause emotional stress, and by adopting new love-based beliefs that liberate us from stress. This type of belief reprogramming can frequently heal chronic headaches in a very short time.

Identifying Fear-Based Beliefs

Most of the headache-causing beliefs we should let go of fit into one of the following patterns.

1. They condemn, judge, criticize or attack someone else.
2. They are unforgiving.
3. They concern the past or future. They cause us to analyze the past and to feel guilt or resentment about something that has already happened. Or they may cause us to worry and become anxious about possible problems that lie in the future.
4. They provoke selfish instincts linked with the body

that arise from fear of lack, and are based on getting and receiving.

5. They cause us to expect a reward for everything we do, or to anticipate fame, wealth, prestige, recognition, praise and other ego-swelling strokes.

6. They cause us to see everything in materialistic terms and to become strongly attached to money and possessions.

7. They cause us to feel discontented and dissatisfied and to crave and want things that are not absolutely essential.

8. They cause us to see difficulties, problems and conflicts in everything.

9. They allow our lives to be run by negative feelings.

10. They confront us with choices when we are tense and emotionally upset. Decisions made when emotionally upset are usually regretted later.

11. They cause us to love a person only if that person meets our conditions.

12. They cause us to compare ourselves with others and to feel dissatisfied.

13. They cause us to compete with and to try to win out over others.

14. They cause us to be rigid and inflexible and to hold strong opinions.

15. They allow us to blame others for the way we are and for what happens to us, creating a convenient victim role for us to play.

16. They cause us to be always concerned with ourselves and to place our own needs ahead of everyone else's.

17. They cause us to fear being alone or doing anything unless we are part of a group.

18. They cause us to magnify molehills into mountains.

19. They cause us to feel insecure, either financially or in relationships.

20. They cause us to feel helpless, hopeless and totally dependent for headache relief on drugs or on passive therapies administered by someone else.

Outdated Beliefs Trigger Destructive Emotions

While beliefs that fit these patterns don't cause headaches directly, they cause us to perceive potentially stressful events in a stressful way.

For example: Julia's sister, acting as executor of their mother's will, keeps for herself a handsome antique clock. Although it wasn't specifically mentioned in the will, Julia feels certain that her mother intended her to have the clock and that her sister was aware of this. As a result, Julia decides that she will never forgive her sister. A few weeks later, she begins to experience migraine headaches. Although she isn't aware of it, whenever she analyzes the past and begins to feel bitter and resentful over the clock, a migraine often appears soon afterwards.

We can easily see that this situation fits into several of the patterns that identify negative beliefs, such as unforgiveness, analyzing the past, wanting things, and so on. Were Julia to let go of these beliefs, in all probability, her migraines would disappear.

To let go of an undesirable belief, you simply *let go of it*. This is made much easier when we replace it with a positive belief. Were Julia to genuinely adopt the positive belief: "I forgive and release forever anyone I have not forgiven, in particular my sister," her migraines would very probably disappear.

Most Headache Sufferers Hold Inappropriate Beliefs

When we continue to hold inappropriate conditioned beliefs—many of them instilled by Madison Avenue brainwashing—we remain locked into a belief system that doesn't work. We spend our time vainly trying to find lasting happiness by buying or doing things which, while they provide a brief glimpse of happiness, only lead in the end to greater dissatisfaction and increasing levels of emotional stress.

Many people believe, for instance, that buying a new car will make them feel happy. It may, for a few days. But then they wake up to the enormous monthly payments they have burdened themselves with and to the huge insurance premiums they must meet. Instead of steering them towards lasting happiness, their negative belief system leads them towards increasing levels of pressure and stress.

A more positive belief system would have steered them towards ceasing to crave a new car. By having their present car repaired instead, they could stay out of debt and remain in a relaxed, positive mind state which would help headache sufferers remain headache-free. Obviously, occasions do arise when a new car, or a new home, may be the soundest investment. But to regard a new car or house as an antidote to unhappiness reveals a serious flaw in a person's belief system.

Positive Beliefs That Liberate Us from Headaches

By adopting the precepts of positivism listed below, we can free ourselves from the majority of headaches.

1. I do and acquire only things which will maintain and deepen my inner peace. I cease craving superficial excitement and stimulation. I realise that lasting happiness comes only from contentment and not from things that I buy, do, eat or drink. When I am content and at ease, my body and mind are calm and relaxed and headaches almost never occur.

2. I forgive and release forever anyone I have not

forgiven—and I rejoice for me. I forgive everyone, everything and every circumstance unconditionally, totally and *right now*!

3. I remain positive all of the time. I accept all the warmth and joy in life but I allow negativity to flow past me and I simply witness it without reacting negatively.

4. I know there is nothing to fear. My headaches will be healed as I let go of fear and as I replace it with unconditional love.

5. I experience only abundance and I am willing to share my abundance with others. For I know that giving and receiving are the same. Whatever I give or lose, I will receive back. (Note: this does not mean you should "loan" money to financially irresponsible people, including members of your own family.)

6. I love everyone unconditionally, including myself, and I accept everyone the way they are without requiring them to change.

7. I am always optimistic, hopeful, cheerful and positive.

8. I completely let go of the past, and with it all guilt and resentment.

9. I have totally ceased to worry about the future. All my fears about the future are imaginary and all my concepts about the future are sheer fantasy. I am a powerful person and I am completely competent to handle whatever the future may bring. Besides, when the future does arrive, it will have become the present.

10. I anticipate tomorrow with enthusiastic expectations. Good things are going to happen to me tomorrow (and also later on today).

11. I live only in the present moment, here and now. Now is the only time there is, for the past is gone and the future is just a fantasy.

12. I choose to enjoy every moment of every day regardless of where I am, what I'm doing, how I'm feeling or who I'm with.

13. I am a hardy person. I am not intimidated by minor discomforts or inconvenience or by physical or mental exertion. I never give up or give in. I always act as if it is impossible to fail.

14. I can heal myself—and I will. I can heal myself from chronic headaches. For healing is to let go of fear and fear-based beliefs. I am completely healed, I can't be sick. Every day in every way I am getting better and better.

15. My birthright is perfect health and perfect health is my normal, natural state.

16. I practice positivism every moment of every day. To be here is joy, to exist is bliss, to be alive is sheer happiness.

17. I act and make choices and decisions only when I am centered, calm and serene. I avoid acting or choosing when I feel emotionally upset.

18. I never use attack thoughts on anyone or anything.

19. I do not expect to be treated with fairness or justice. Both exist only in the eye of a beholder.

20. I accept complete responsibility for my life and for everything that happens to me.

21. I recognize that absolute material security is unattainable. Yet I also know that I will always have what I want when I need it.

22. I always tell the complete truth and I reveal my deepest feelings. I never repress or conceal a negative feeling.

23. I am one with every living thing. I never see myself as separate from others.

24. I always act without anticipating results, without seeking the fruits or rewards of my actions. I act selflessly while expressing love and compassion.

25. I see only the best in everyone including myself.

26. I am content to be wherever I am here and now. I

always have everything I need to enjoy the present moment. Therefore my needs and wants are few.

27. I have no desire for praise, attention, fame or recognition or to appear publicly important. I will not do anything merely to win the approval of others. I refuse to experience pride. I always practice humility.

28. I share the good and success that comes to others without any hint of envy. I never compare myself with others or with their accomplishments or possessions. As a result, I am liberated from envy.

29. I can only win when everyone wins.

Restructuring Your Belief System with Positivism

To put cognitive positivism to work, all you need do is to accept, one by one, each of the 29 positive beliefs. Starting with number 1, study it until you have accepted it completely. Don't go past number 2 until you actually have chosen to forgive everyone whom you believe may have caused you harm at some time.

By the simple act of mentally accepting each positive belief, you will also be releasing its opposite belief, the inappropriate conditioned belief that caused you to perceive events as stressful and that, in turn, caused your headaches.

For example, past events may have conditioned you to believe that the only way to have security is to build a fortress of money. While it may still be prudent to provide for a possible rainy day and for retirement, it is much more appropriate to recognize that life offers an unlimited abundance of love and goodness and that we need no longer continue to look at everything from a position of lack.

Behavioral Medicine's Most Powerful Healing Tool

A rapidly growing body of facts revealed by the leading edge of scientific research is offering intriguing evidence of the mind's healing power. Literally dozens of studies in immunity research are strongly confirming that negative beliefs, thoughts, feelings and attitudes suppress our immunity while positive beliefs, thoughts, emotions and attitudes enhance our immunity. Since our immunocompetence is as closely associated with the fight-or-flight response as our headaches, it follows that the same negative emotions that suppress immunity also cause headaches.

Cognitive positivism evolved out of the pioneering work of such top medical researchers as oncologists Bernie Siegel and O. Carl Simonton, cardiologists Herbert Benson and Dean Ornish, David T. Burns, M.D. of the University of Pennsylvania, Joan Borysenko, Ph.D. of Harvard Medical School's Body-Mind Clinic, Gerald Jampolsky, M.D., originator of attitudinal healing, and Paul Pearsall, Ph.D. of Detroit's Sinai Hospital.

The fact that cognitive positivism has been endorsed by highly accredited doctors from top-ranking university medical schools testifies to its effectiveness. It is the *only* therapy that stops the headache process dead in its tracks before it can even initiate Stage 1. No drug in existence works at this level.

By adopting each of the 29 new positive beliefs, we rid ourselves of negative thoughts. Without a negative thought, we cannot experience a negative feeling. And without a negative feeling we cannot become depressed, fearful, unhappy, angry, anxious, resentful, guilty, or frustrated nor can we experience any kind of downer.

When we deliberately adopt love-based beliefs and thoughts, we begin to see the world as a loving, friendly, non-threatening place. Our focus is on the immediate here and now. By zeroing in on the present moment, we are able to let go of the past and its guilts and resentments, and we realize that whatever the future may hold, we are perfectly capable and confident of being able to handle it.

We begin to see everyone as our brother and sister, and we begin to accept everyone the way they are, and we ask no changes of anyone. We begin to experience a wonderful feeling of oneness with every person and living thing. The concept of feeling separate from other people disappears and with it, any feelings of loneliness.

Right now, at this moment, we realize that there is nothing we need or want. As a result, we feel content and we begin to experience inner peace. We suddenly find we are no longer condemning or judging others. This, then, leads us to forgive everyone whom we once believed had harmed us in some way.

We become almost completely liberated from emotional stress, and from all stress-related diseases and dysfunctions. And somewhere in the process our headaches disappear.

10 The Lifestyle Approach

Headache *prevention* is the theme of the lifestyle approach. And we can achieve headache freedom by assimilating into our lifestyle all behaviors and beliefs that minimize headaches and by dropping all risk factors that intensify headaches.

All too many chronic headache sufferers have built a lifestyle centered around their pain. Gradually, by taking endless medication, they have destroyed their sleep habits, become fearful of physical exertion, developed a poor posture, and acquired habitual use of proven headache triggers, all creating a vicious circle which merely exacerbates headache pain.

We can break this pain-centered lifestyle by taking the first steps towards a headache-free lifestyle. By simply dropping one headache-provoking habit and replacing it with a health-building habit, we can create a powerful change in attitude that immediately motivates us to begin breaking all headache-reinforcing habits.

Most habits, foods, beliefs and migraine triggers that

provoke headaches have been described in earlier chapters. The purpose of this chapter is to review the remainder.

☐ Anti-Headache Technique #18: Live a Headache-Free Lifestyle

Stop Smoking

Not only is smoking a suicidal, health-wrecking habit but it is one of the major causes of all types of headaches. No one can feel completely safe from headaches until he or she has quit smoking for good.

Space prevents our giving a complete stop-smoking strategy. But we do know that more people are addicted to nicotine than to all street and prescription drugs combined, and that smoking is as addictive as heroin or cocaine.

Nicotine stimulates production of beta-endorphin and certain neurotransmitters that cause alertness, arousal, a feeling of pleasure, and freedom from pain and anxiety.

What smokers fail to realize is that regular daily exercise, such as a brisk five-mile walk, provides exactly the same level of alertness, arousal, and a feeling of pleasure, and freedom from pain and anxiety as does smoking, all without the health risks of smoking. (All smokers should have their doctor's permission before taking up exercise.)

Additionally, most stop-smoking authorities advise switching from smoking to chewing a nicotine-based gum like Nicorettes. The goal is then to gradually break your addiction to the gum—a task made much easier when you exercise daily.

You are also advised to enroll in a non-commercial stop smoking clinic sponsored by the American Cancer Society, American Lung Association, American Heart Association or the Seventh-Day Adventists. To complete your program, you should have your doctor issue you an absolute and strongly worded ultimatum to quit smoking immediately.

The many other steps you can take are described in books or are taught in the clinics. Don't be afraid of gaining a few pounds. To equal the health risk of smoking, you would have to be 120 pounds overweight. And if you do slip up, begin to quit smoking again *immediately*. Don't take a second cigarette. A single slip won't wreck your intentions.

Maintain Regular Sleep Patterns

Sleeping with your head under the covers permits an oversupply of carbon dioxide to accumulate in blood vessels. Carbon dioxide is a powerful blood vessel dilator and migraine trigger.

Anyone who sleeps for under five hours or for more than ten hours each night also increases risk of migraine. Fatigue due to lack of sleep is another well-known migraine trigger. Thus it's important to maintain regular sleep patterns throughout the week. Get up at the same time every day and avoid oversleeping on weekend mornings.

Those prone to tension headaches should avoid sleeping on the stomach. It forcibly turns your head to one side, creating muscular tension that could easily set off a headache. If you sleep on your back, place a small pillow beneath the neck to prevent the head from being tilted either backwards or forwards. Likewise, if you sleep on your side, avoid slumping the head forward.

Special "cervical pillows" are available, designed to allow the neck to relax while sleeping on the back or side. You may also obtain a horseshoe-shaped pillow stuffed with a gel pack which you can freeze in the refrigerator and place under the head and neck to relieve a headache. Called the Suboccipital Ice Pillow, it is available from SPF Distributors, 1545 North Verdugo Road, Glendale CA 91208. This mention does not imply our endorsement.

Use Your Diary to Identify Headache Triggers

Careful diary-keeping is a great help in identifying the exact nature of tension or migraine headache triggers. Women should include exact dates on which menstruation begins and ends. After three months, you should begin to see a pattern which can help to identify migraine triggers and to avoid them.

Diary-keeping coupled with careful observation also can help identify tension headache triggers. For example, you may find that it is not typing that causes your headache but the way you sit or slouch over the typewriter. Or it could be due to inadequate lighting. Identifying and avoiding headache triggers has brought relief to many.

Here is a brief rundown of the principal categories of headache triggers.

PHYSICAL AND ENVIRONMENTAL TRIGGERS

Smog-containing sulphur dioxide, commonly emitted from refineries, steel and paper mills or fertilizer plants, has been scientifically confirmed as a common migraine trigger. Fumes and odors from soap, detergent, perfume, after-shave lotion, and household chemicals and pesticides, when inhaled in an enclosed room, can set off migraine in some people.

Other common environmental triggers include glaring or flickering lights or bright outdoor sunshine (wear sunglasses and a hat with a brim).

Stale air in offices and rooms, especially if smoke-filled, is a potential headache trigger. Others include: odorless carbon monoxide leaks from car exhausts or heating equipment; rapid decreases in barometric pressure; wearing a swim mask or goggles—this can set off a headache one to two hours later; sudden weather changes, especially onset of a hot, dry wind.

Loud, jarring noises keep the body continually stressed, while a constant noise prevents relaxation. Temporary headaches due to high elevation are also common among mountain hikers and climbers. Usually mild, the headaches customarily affect the entire head. Occasionally, an altitude headache is confined to one side, and can become as severe as a migraine. Altitude headaches normally disappear on descending.

Long distance flights, especially from east to west, can trigger migraine in susceptible persons. To help avoid headaches when flying, drink frequent glasses of water, avoid alcohol, eat lightly, sit in an aisle seat so that you can stand up and stretch, and rest upon arrival. OTC painkillers are freely available on most flights.

POOR POSTURE TRIGGERS

Abrupt changes of posture can trigger tension headaches. Avoid cradling a phone under your chin for more than a few minutes. Sit up straight and keep the head erect and the shoulders low while using the phone. Whether standing, sitting or lying, keep the shoulders *down*. Avoid hunching them up around the ears.

Avoid slouching or slumping at any time, especially while watching TV. Place the TV screen at the same level as your eyes and straight in front so that you avoid looking down or turning your head. Get up and walk around at least once per hour, roll and rotate the shoulders and neck, and pull the shoulder blades together several times.

Avoid working overhead with your arms and hands raised for long periods. Use a stepladder instead. Don't permit your head to slump or hang forward. Always sit and stand tall, straight and upright. When sitting at a desk or working at a bench, change positions every fifteen minutes. Breathe through the nose, keep your tongue relaxed, and avoid grinding the teeth. Also avoid shallow breathing. Inhale fully and fill the bottoms of your lungs at each breath.

Reading or working in a poor light is a common cause of headaches. Use a bulb with a minimum power of 60 watts directed down over your shoulder. We used a 250-watt soft white light bulb mounted overhead while writing this book. Fluorescent lighting is even better. The older you are, the stronger the light you should have.

Poor posture while slouched over and reading in bed can also contribute to tension headache. Avoid reading in bed with your head propped up on pillows. Instead, sit upright in bed with a pillow under your knees to prevent pressure on muscles in the lower back. Always sleep on a pillow. Sleeping without a pillow causes more blood to flow to the head, setting the stage for a migraine attack.

TIME PRESSURE STRESS AS HEADACHE TRIGGER

People whose lives are filled with deadlines and pressures commonly suffer from tension or migraine headaches. Most of us can slow the pace of our lives by letting go of nonessential activities such as volunteer work, and by turning down all demands on our time that create added pressure.

Almost all of us are able to put the brakes on a busy helter-skelter lifestyle so that we have more time to work, play, eat and relax at a leisurely pace. With careful planning, we can usually rearrange our lives to take time out each day for fun, games and socializing.

Build up a week's income in reserve so that you don't have to stand and wait in line at the bank or supermarket during the Friday afternoon crush. Go on Tuesday instead. Shop early in the morning or after 7 P.M., when supermarkets are often empty. Plan activities well in advance so that you start out in plenty of time, especially for work. Find the location of new places you must visit on a street map before you leave home. And prevent rush by doing only one thing at a time.

Although Americans tend to glorify the automobile, and a car is essential in most locations, driving under today's high-speed conditions is far from pleasant. Several studies have concluded that car ownership actually lowers the quality of most peoples' lives. It places a severe strain on our finances, while driving and maintaining a car can be one of the most stressful aspects of modern living. Among other things, it can entrap us into becoming a chauffeur for our children.

Try to minimize driving on freeways or in congested traffic. For short trips, use a bicycle or walk instead. And you can help reduce automobile stress by keeping your older car instead of buying a new one, and by spending as little time in the car as you can.

Try to avoid a sudden letdown from stress as you end a hectic week on Friday afternoon and find yourself in an inertia vacuum on Saturday morning. This situation can frequently provoke a migraine, especially if your job entails long days of listening, talking, telephoning and making decisions.

The answer is to even out your work week, and to try and spread your tasks and work load evenly over each day. Most of us could gradually phase out a crowded schedule by pacing ourselves differently. Many migraineurs create unnecessary stress by their inability to live with an uncompleted task. The solution, of course, is to never be afraid to postpone completion of a nonessential task.

Above all, we need to learn to live life for today and to enjoy every moment for what it's worth.

About the Author

Norman D. Ford is a medical researcher, a self-help author and an expert in holistic therapies. He has written for *Prevention* and *Bestways* and other well-known health magazines and has lectured extensively to health groups and organizations. Ford has authored more than forty books in the fields of retirement, leisure and health. He practices what he preaches and his lifestyle is built around the Whole Person health practices described in this book. An avid hiker, bicyclist, swimmer and vegetarian, Ford lives in the Texas Hill Country. He is an accredited member of the American Medical Writers Association.

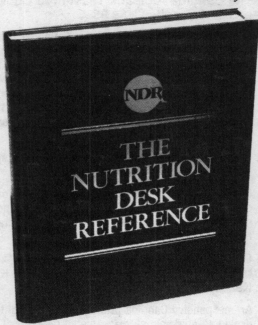